EXECUTIVE FITNESS

Other books available in this series

- COPING WITH EXECUTIVE STRESS
- EXECUTIVE NUTRITION AND DIET

EXECUTIVE FITNESS

Executive Health Examiners

Richard E. Winter, M.D.
Series Editor

McGraw-Hill Book Company

New York   St. Louis   San Francisco   Auckland   Bogotá   Guatemala   Hamburg
Johannesburg   Lisbon   London   Madrid   Mexico   Montreal   New Delhi   Panama
Paris   San Juan   São Paulo   Singapore   Sidney   Tokyo   Toronto

The Author

Marc Leepson has authored numerous articles on health and exercise for some of America's leading publications, including THE NEW YORK TIMES, WASHINGTON POST, CHICAGO TRIBUNE, CHRISTIAN SCIENCE MONITOR, and SMITHSONIAN MAGAZINE.

EXECUTIVE FITNESS

Copyright © 1983 by McGraw-Hill, Inc. All rights reserved. Printed in the United States of America. Except as permitted under the United States Copyright Act of 1976, no part of this publication may be reproduced or distributed in any form or by any means, or stored in a data base or retrieval system, without the prior written permission of the publisher.

1234567890 DODO 898765432

ISBN 0-07-019863-2

This book was set in Zapf Book Light by Progressive Typographers; the editors were Robert P. McGraw and Maggie Schwarz; the production supervisor was Jeanne Skahan; the designer was Murray Fleminger. R. R. Donnelley & Sons Company was printer and binder.

See Acknowledgments on page 199.
Copyrights included on this page by reference.

Library of Congress Cataloging in Publication Data
Main Entry under title:

Executive fitness.

   (Executive health series)
   Includes index.
   1. Exercise. 2. Physical fitness.
3. Executives—Health programs. I. Executive
Health Examiners (U.S.) II. Series.
GV481.E96   613.7'044   82-15206
ISBN 0-07-019863-2   AACR2

Executive Health Examiners

Richard E. Winter, M.D.	*Chairman*

William S. Wanago, M.D.	*Senior Vice President of Medical Affairs*
John A. Rossa, M.D.	*Director, New York Executive Clinic*
Allyn Kidwell, M.D.	*Director, Morristown Executive Clinic*
John M. Hill, M.D.	*Director, Stamford Executive Clinic*
Gazanfer Alkaya, M.D.	*Director, New York Stock Exchange Clinic*
Charles Ulrich, M.D.	*Director, Ambulatory Health Service Clinic*
Neil Crane, M.D.	*Director, EHE Washington Bureau*
Julio Rivera, M.D.	*Director, Occupational Medical Service, NIH Clinic*
Barbara Wasserman, M.D.	*Director, Clinical Medicine, NIH Clinic*
John Foulke, M.D.	*Director, NASA Goddard Clinic*
Richard Ross, M.D.	*Director, Fairchild Republic Clinic*
Gitanjali Mukerjee, M.D.	*Director, Spofford Detention Center, Medical Service*
William McBride, M.D.	*Director, NASA Dryden Research Center, Medical Service*
Fred Block, M.D.	*Director, Chemical Bank Clinic*
Frank Marzullo, M.D.	*Director, Bank of New York Clinic*
Donna M. Hartl, M.D.	*Director, Johnson & Higgins Clinic*
Riska Platt, M.S., R.D.	*Director, Nutrition Programs*
Steven Tay, M.D.	*Associate Director, New York Executive Clinic*
Jack Goldman, M.D.	*Associate Director, New York Stock Exchange Clinic*
Socrates Fotiu, M.D.	*Associate Director, NASA Goddard Clinic*
Stanley Craig, M.D.	*Radiology*
Stanley Halprin, M.D.	*Cardiology*
Lawrence Koblenz, M.D.	*Gastroenterology*
Stephen Krasnica, M.D.	*Cardiology*
Mauro Mecca, M.D.	*Internal Medicine*
Bernard Nemoitin, M.D.	*Proctology*
Jasu Sanghvi, M.D.	*Gynecology*
Erasmo Sturla, M.D.	*Endocrinology*
Sidney Wanderman, M.D.	*Proctology*
Mel Weinstein, M.D.	*Internal Medicine*
Madeleine Steele	*Project Coordinator*

CONTENTS

PREFACE

Twenty-five years ago, in one of our preeminent medical research centers, there resided a group of very special laboratory animals. Challenged constantly, forced to make decisions and to act under pressure, they were the "executive monkeys." In one famous experiment, two monkeys were placed side-by-side in chairs equipped to give electric shocks. One of the monkeys—and only one—could prevent the shocks to both itself and its partner by pressing a lever. Under the psychological stress of being responsible for pressing the lever, this executive monkey developed duodenal ulcers.

The close correlation of behavior patterns in animals and humans has been thoroughly documented by scientific research. It has been shown that information obtained from animal research can be successfully applied to human research and experience. The study of animal behavior, for example, can result in a better understanding of the behavior of the individuals who go out each day to lead our governments, industries, and unions.

Few of us have ever watched chimpanzees in their natural habitat, the jungles of Africa. If we could observe these animals, we would see that they wander around, nibbling a few nuts here, a few berries there, eating continuously in small amounts. What they do *not* do is neglect eating for long periods and then pour raw alcohol onto the tender mucosal linings of their stomachs. They do *not* smoke several cigarettes, and thereby increase the outpouring of hydrochloric acid. They do *not* then consume large quantities of food, try to exist on insufficient sleep, and undergo rapid changes in environment. If they did, they would very likely suffer the same fate as a number of American executives under observation at a major research center who, possessing one or more of these habits, died before the study could be completed.

Medical science has accumulated an enormous amount of significant data from studies on animals and humans. As always, though, the important task is putting that knowledge to use in practical ways that can most benefit humankind. EXECUTIVE HEALTH EXAMINERS was founded more than twenty years ago for the primary purpose of making medical knowledge available to a particular group—executives. Over the years our medical staff has examined executives from every kind of business and profession and at every level. From this vast experience it has become apparent to us that these executives—men and women alike—are often *simultaneously* exposed to all the life-threatening habits that chimpanzees naturally avoid. And it is this circumstance that, in our opinion, makes executives unique. Other groups are, of course, subjected to some of the same threats to their health, but, in our experience, only in the executive lifestyle do these threats converge at the same time.

The conviction that executives are unique, that their lifestyles are different and therefore their health needs special, led us to prepare a series of books specifically for executives. In these volumes we combine solid medical fact with our years of professional experience to provide practical, proven approaches to solving health problems. Each volume deals with an area of health where executives are especially vulnerable. COPING WITH EXECUTIVE STRESS provides the most current medical information on stress and its effect on both the mind and body to show executives how to recognize and cope with stress in executive life. EXECUTIVE NUTRITION AND DIET is a commonsense program for nutrition and diet that has been highly successful for thousands of executives. All the special problems of executive lifestyle are dealt with in this basic, balanced discussion of sound nutritional habits and healthy diet. EXECUTIVE FITNESS is a flexible, workable exercise program designed for busy executives. Within a basic format, it offers a wide variety of exercise options, all of which are certain to result in increased stamina and productivity.

There is no question that the demands of executive life make good health maintenance difficult. Having guided hundreds of thousands of executives to positive and lasting changes in their lifestyle, however, we know that the habits of eating properly, exercising regularly and coping with stress can be successfully acquired. The volumes in this series offer sound information gained from long and specific experience with executives. We view these books as a kind of survival kit for executives. It is our hope that they will enable every executive to enjoy a longer, healthier, more productive and satisfying life.

Richard E. Winter, M.D.

Richard E. Winter, M.D.
Chairman

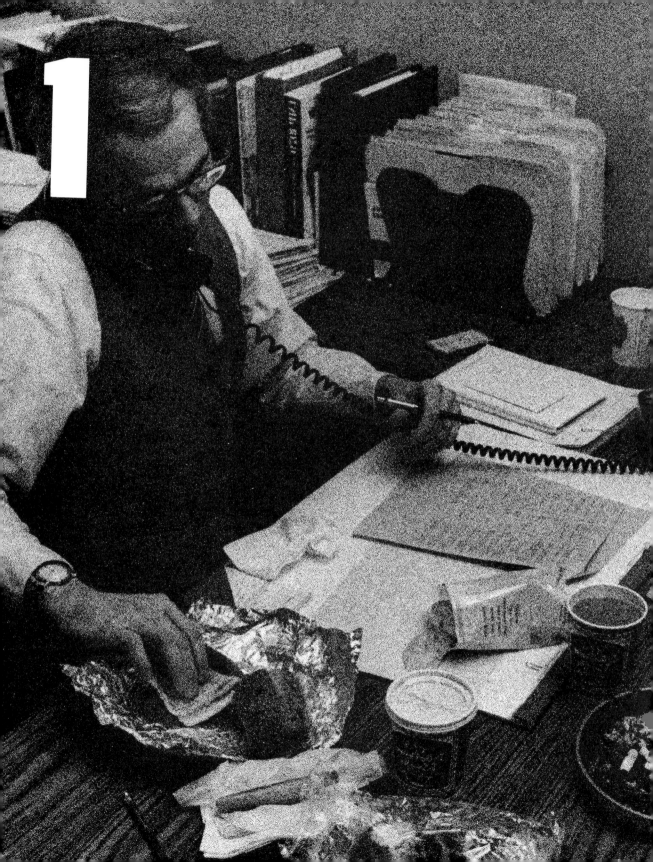

WHY EVERY EXECUTIVE NEEDS TO EXERCISE

Let us face it—executives are sitting for most of their workdays, and in the evenings and on weekends as well. Think about your own daily schedule. Does it go something like this? Up at 6:30 A.M., with time only for a shower and a cup of coffee before you are off to work. Then a frustrating 45-minute drive through rush-hour traffic to work. You park in a garage and take the elevator up to the office. Then comes an 8-hour day or more, stuck for the most part behind a desk, and then another drive home. After supper you sit down in your favorite easy chair in front of the television set.

The routine is the same for 5 or even 6 days a week. Sometimes on the weekend you work in the yard, raking leaves, cutting the grass, and so on. You play tennis occasionally. You travel regularly, spending most of that time on airplanes, in meetings, and in hotel rooms.

If your life follows this pattern, you are living an almost totally sedentary existence, an existence that medical scientists now believe is a contributing factor to heart disease and to a host of other disabling and potentially deadly diseases.

A sedentary executive lifestyle was rare 150 years ago. Before the industrial age, nearly everyone in the United States depended on physical movement for food and shelter. Just a century ago, dawn-to-dusk working hours were prevalent

A sedentary lifestyle can be a contributing factor to heart disease and other ailments.

not only on farms and in factories but in many businesses as well. Until the mid-nineteenth century the only people who did not have exhausting workdays were the wealthy in the large eastern cities and in the south. For most Americans the only leisure time came on Sunday, when they welcomed a day of rest called for by the biblical injunction to rest on the seventh day of the week.

In the post-Civil War era, as the nation became more industrialized, large numbers of Americans for the first time no longer had to expend themselves physically to attain the necessities of life. By the end of the 1920s, working conditions had eased to the point where the 8-hour day with a half day off on Saturday had become standard. The real impetus for shorter working hours came during the prosperous economy in the years following World War II.

Today there are few professions that provide adequate amounts of physical exercise during the course of an average workday. This, of course, includes almost every executive job. Even construction and manufacturing jobs often fall short of providing the vigorous physical exertion they once required. In 1850, about one-third of the energy used in farms and factories was provided by human muscle. Today the figure is down to one-half of 1 percent.

In our advanced industrialized society, even construction workers can use sophisticated machinery to save a good deal, though not all, of the physical effort once demanded by their jobs. The same is true with most factory jobs. "Everything is mechanized in factories so workers rarely move from one spot, and never lift anything above their waists or below their knees," reports Guy Reiff, professor of physical education at the University of Michigan, who studied 160 factory workers for 10 years to measure how much on-the-job exercise they received.[1]

The Sedentary Lifestyle

Richard O. Keelor, the longtime director of program development for the President's Council on Physical Fitness and Sports, has a cogent description for the typical sedentary executive lifestyle. He calls it "habitual inactivity." Keelor has identified two of the most serious health hazards in the American workplace. They are not asbestos and coal dust but the desk and the swivel chair, which deprive working men and women of the opportunity to exercise. Today's typical office job, Keelor says, requires "less exertion than a hot shower."[2]

The consequences of habitual inactivity are not pleasant to contemplate; they include degeneration of the muscular, respiratory, and cardiovascular systems.

Many scientists now believe that sedentary work and living habits are not compatible with the design of the human body. They contend that the body's muscular, respiratory, and circulatory systems not only need, but were designed specifically for, participation in regular vigorous movements. Depriving the body of regular vigorous exercise can therefore cause these systems to degenerate.

James Nora, M.D., director of preventive cardiology at the University of Colorado School of Medicine, calls the sedentary life the "nonphysical lifestyle." Dr. Nora describes the effects of this lifestyle on the body in the following manner: "The less physical work you do, the less physical work your body becomes capable of doing. And the converse is also true: The more physical work you do (up to defined limits), the more you become able to do. . . . Demand little and you get little. Demand a lot and you get a lot. That's the homeostatic wisdom of the body."[3]

[1] "The Fitness Mania," *U.S. News & World Report*, February 27, 1978, p. 38.
[2] From a speech to the Blue Shield annual program conference, Chicago, October 4, 1976.
[3] James Jackson Nora, *The Whole Heart Book* (New York: Holt, Rinehart and Winston, 1980), p. 156.

Demanding little of the body can lead to degeneration, which in turn can cause heart disease, stroke, hypertension, and premature aging. In short, depriving the body of regular exercise also deprives it of health and vitality. As Keelor says:

> Experiments have shown that prolonged bed rest, or chair rest, can transform a robust young man into a feeble fellow with weak muscles and the unsteady gait of an old man. Sedentary work and living habits have the same debilitative effects, though they are slower to develop—and more insidious because they are so often mistaken for the normal ravages of time.

As the Blue Cross/Blue Shield publication "A Very Simple Guide to Help You Feel Better" (1980) puts it, "We are not only beneficiaries of the industrial, technological, scientific and electronic revolution: we are victims of it."

Exercise as an Antidote to the Sedentary Lifestyle

A growing number of medical authorities now believe that exercise can be an antidote to the sedentary lifestyle. In fact, Executive Health Examiners sees exercise as a form of preventive medicine that almost always leads to better physical and mental health. We have found that a complete, balanced exercise program, when combined with a healthy diet and lifestyle, can contribute to the prevention of many diseases, including the most prevalent and dangerous physical problem facing executives: cardiovascular disease.

Executive Health Examiners has found that no one—not even the most deskbound executive—has to suffer the con-

Scientists now believe that sedentary work and living habits are not compatible with the design of the human body.

sequences of the sedentary lifestyle. We have devised a preventive medicine prescription that almost any executive can follow. It is a three-part system designed to eliminate or greatly lessen the risk factors associated with the disease executives are most likely to face. The first step after checking with your doctor is to begin a regular, balanced exercise program along the lines of the ones we recommend in detail beginning in Chapter 2. We also urge our patients to adopt sensible eating habits. We recommend cutting down on foods with high fat, cholesterol, sugar, and salt content, while eating more fresh vegetables, fruit, and whole grains. Finally, we urge our clients to make significant changes in their daily lives: to stop smoking cigarettes and abusing alcohol and drugs and to learn how to cope with mental stress. Exercise alone is not the answer; all three factors must interact.

We cannot guarantee that a regular physical exercise program will prolong your life or provide ironclad protection against heart disease or other health problems. However, hundreds of scientific tests in recent years have shown that those who exercise are indeed healthier and have a lower incidence of heart disease than those who do not.

Some of the most dramatic evidence was presented in 1977 by Ralph S. Paffenbarger, Jr., M.D., epidemiologist at Stanford University Medical Center. Dr. Paffenbarger and his colleagues spent two decades examining the physical condition and exercise patterns of thousands of men in two groups with widely different lifestyles: 6300 San Francisco longshoremen and 36,500 men who entered Harvard University between 1916 and 1950. The study of the longshoremen revealed that those who engaged in regular patterns of hard physical work were only half as likely to succumb to a sudden-death heart attack as those with less physically demanding jobs. Moreover, the number of heart attacks among all the longshoremen began to increase in the early 1950s after the introduction of mechanization and the use of shipping containers that considerably lightened their workload.

The study of the Harvard men, whose ages ranged from 35 to 75, yielded similar results. The men who expended at least 2000 calories a week through strenuous exercise such as running and swimming had one-third fewer heart attacks than their peers who led sedentary lives. The study also revealed that those who engaged only in light exercise such as bowling or golf were about as likely to have heart attacks as those who got little or no exercise.

Paffenbarger's conclusion:

"Given their contrasts in education, occupation, leisure activities, and ways of living, both study populations have repeated associations of lower heart attack risk with increased energy output. The currently more active persons have lower heart attack risks within their own populations. On this point perhaps it becomes permissible to generalize to other populations or particularize to an individual. Risk of heart attack is increased if physical activity is reduced below favorable levels, and risk is lowered if adequate exercise is maintained."[4]

It is important to keep in mind that the Paffenbarger studies have not proved conclusively that exercise prevents heart attacks or prolongs life. The tests strongly suggest that this is so, but science still cannot answer the pivotal question about those who exercise: Are they healthier because they exercise, or do they tend to exercise because they are healthy?

Exercise as Preventive Medicine

Nevertheless, Executive Health Examiners heartily recommends exercise as a preventive medicine technique, and we believe it can help nearly everyone become healthier, stronger, and more resistant to disease. Although science has yet to prove beyond doubt that exercise is 100 percent effective in prolonging life and preventing heart problems, the evidence is overwhelming that this is so. For the vast majority of executives, exercise is a prudent and beneficial undertaking. Even medical scientists who do not believe that exercise programs can reduce the risk of cardiovascular disease still recommend that most people take part in regular exercise regimens.

Here are the conclusions of an American College of Car-

<hr />

[4] Ralph S. Paffenbarger, Jr., et al., "Current Exercise and Heart Attack Risk," *Cardiac Rehabilitation*, Summer 1979, p. 4.

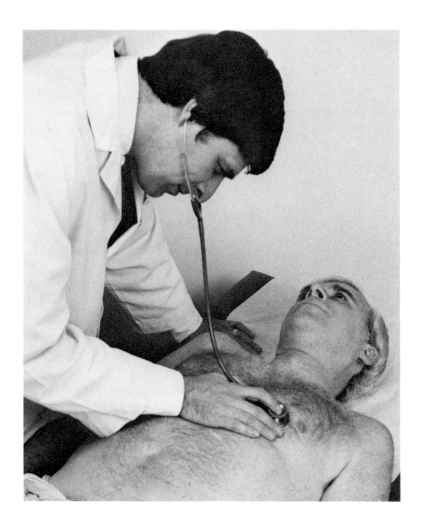

diology-sponsored task force on the Prevention of Coronary
Heart Disease, chaired by Robert S. Eliot, M.D., director of
the University of Nebraska Medical Center's Cardiovascular
Center:

> Although exercise programs have received a great deal of pub-
> licity, their benefits in reducing cardiovascular disease are still
> uncertain. Scientific evidence from many sources suggests
> that people who are vigorously active have less heart disease,
> have an increased sense of well being and are less depressed
> and anxious than are people who are sedentary. If people en-
> tering an exercise program also stop smoking cigarettes, alter
> their diet, lower their body-weight, reduce serum lipids [cho-

lesterol-like fatty deposits in the bloodstream] and bring levels of arterial blood pressure to ideal values, then they probably lower their risk for cardiovascular disease.[5]

There may be some equivocation in that statement, but the message is clear. Exercise can do most people no harm, and there is a very real possibility that it will help prevent a heart attack. At the very least, exercise will help you look and feel better physically and feel better mentally.

Getting the Right Kind of Exercise

One of the first questions EHE doctors ask a patient about to take a physical examination is, "Do you get any exercise?" About 75 percent of the executives we examine say, "Yes, but I don't think I get enough." They are usually right. Not only do they not get enough exercise, they usually do not get the right kind. Consider these two examples:

The vice president of a New Jersey savings and loan association, on days when he feels especially chipper, will do his exercise routine in the morning before showering. The routine, which he has been doing on and off (mostly off) since high school, consists of situps and pushups. On a good day he can do 35 pushups and 100 situps. When he is through with the routine, he is panting and sweating but happy. The situps flatten his stomach, and the pushups build his arm and chest muscles.

A female executive of a sporting goods chain climbs the stairs at work instead of using the elevator, walks several blocks to and from her commuter train, and works around the house on weekends. That is the extent of her regular exercising.

These two executives know they are not getting enough exercise; they told EHE doctors that they were not feeling exactly "right." One of the most common complaints we hear is that an executive feels tired in the late afternoon and evening or even in the morning after awakening. One 39-year-old vice president of a men's clothing chain put it this

---

[5] Robert S. Eliot, et al., "The Physician in the Work Setting," *The American Journal of Cardiology*, March 1981, p. 50.

Exercise can do most people no harm, and there is a very real possibility that it will prevent a heart attack.

way: "My back's been bothering me lately. I'm lethargic, and I wake up in the morning still tired. I don't quite know how to put my finger on it. Eating, sleeping, and so on are all okay. I'm not having any trouble with the family. The job's all right. I just don't particularly feel quite right. I guess I'm getting older."

That man may be getting older, but he does not necessarily have to feel the aging process so acutely. His lack of energy, as with the other two executives who complained that they did not quite feel right, is due to the fact that he does not get the correct type of exercise. The irregular, unbalanced types of exercise that all three executives take part in do not compensate for the habitual inactivity involved in their everyday lives. In spite of the sporadic exercising, their bodies are stagnating. They need to get involved in regular, balanced exercise programs.

Exercising to Ameliorate Risk Factors

Cardiologists and the members of the American Heart Association have identified the probable causes, or risk factors, which they believe are associated with diseases of the heart and blood vessels such as heart attacks and strokes. The risk factors fall into two general categories: those which can be controlled and those which cannot. The uncontrollable risk factors are age, sex, family history, and susceptibility to diseases such as diabetes. The controllable risk factors are a sedentary lifestyle, cigarette smoking, obesity, high blood pressure, high cholesterol levels, and modification of "Type A" behavior. See the list of coronary risk factors.

Executive Health Examiners has found that every one of

CORONARY RISK FACTORS

Controllable	Uncontrollable
High cholesterol level	Family history of heart disease
High blood pressure	Age
Smoking	Sex
Unmodified Type A behavior	Inherited susceptibility to diseases such as diabetes
Obesity	
Sedentary lifestyle	

the controllable risk factors associated with cardiovascular disease can be mitigated through exercise. We advise most executives who come to us with these risk factors to begin exercise programs after first consulting a physician. In fact, anyone over 35 should have a complete physical examination including a stress test before embarking on any exercise program. With proper medical guidance, most executives can easily undertake an exercise regimen that probably will reduce the risk factors for cardiovascular disease.

We have found that executives who need regular exercise fall into three broad categories: those who get no exercise; those who get some, but the wrong kind; and those who require reduction in cardiovascular risk factors. What about healthy executives who do not have any risk factors or physical complaints? Should they exercise? Many executives seem to fit in that category. After reviewing health statistics on executives, Joseph LaDou, medical director of a California industrial clinic, concluded that because many large businesses and corporations stress physical fitness for their executives, "the stereotype of unhealthy executive is false." LaDou says that "as a group, executives are healthier than other workers."[6] This may be true. Executive Health Examiners nevertheless advises healthy executives to embark on a balanced exercise program even if they show no signs of risk and have no specific physical complaints.

A New York City account executive who came to Executive Health Examiners recently for a physical examination provides a good example. We found that this 46-year-old

[6] Joseph LaDou, *The Executive*, March 1979.

man was only about 5 pounds overweight. He did not smoke, had low cholesterol and blood pressure levels, and overall was in good health. He had no coronary risk factors, yet we still recommended that he undertake an exercise program.

When he asked us why, we told him that there are several important benefits to be derived from an exercise program besides the amelioration of coronary risk factors. For one thing, we have found that people involved in exercise programs seem to sharpen themselves mentally. They are able to concentrate better at work, and consequently they become more productive and effective on the job.

Building Reserve Strength

There is also the important factor of building reserve strength. A balanced exercise program provides cardiovascular conditioning and helps strengthen and tone the muscles, thus building bodily strength. This can prove very beneficial when the unexpected happens and you need to call on your reserves. If you break a leg, for instance, and are forced to get around on crutches, you will be able to handle that physically demanding task more easily if you have reserve strength, which will allow you to function at a relatively normal level. Or you might have to dash from one end of a large airport terminal to the other, carrying a heavy suitcase. Reserve strength from exercise (plus that surge of adrenaline) will go a long way toward getting you through the physical emergency without placing undue strain on your heart, and you might well catch that plane.

If the points in the box sound familiar, then you probably

Every one of the controllable risk factors associated with cardiovascular disease can be mitigated through exercise.

ARE YOU A TYPE A?

Does this sound like you?

- You are a very competitive person, not only at work but at play.
- You like to go straight to the heart of every matter, and you do not rest until whatever you are working on is completed.
- You hate waiting in line for anything.
- You despise getting caught in a traffic jam and waiting in line at the bank.
- You are conscious of time at every moment of the day, and you often lose your temper when something unexpected happens to disrupt your carefully prearranged schedule.
- You are always doing at least two things at once, racing against a deadline to finish both and move on to two more things.
- You never seem to have enough time to complete the many tasks of your business day.

have a "Type A" personality. Many cardiologists believe that this type of personality greatly enhances a person's chances of developing heart disease. Two California cardiologists, Drs. Meyer Friedman and Ray H. Rosenman, began studying the link between Type A personalities and heart disease in 1960. After a decade of research involving 35,000 people, they found that 70 percent of the people they studied who developed heart disease had Type A personalities.

Executive Health Examiners has found that exercise is one way to lessen harmful Type A personality traits. Exercising in a noncompetitive manner tends to calm the mind and reduce stress, and there is an additional residual effect. A complete, balanced exercise program can help an executive long after the exercise period is finished by calming the mind and enabling the executive to cope more effectively. You can handle stress much more easily with a refreshed and relaxed mind and body.

Being physically fit also can help you cope with disease more effectively. We have found that our well-conditioned patients who experience unexpected illnesses seem to have a significantly easier time tolerating disease. Whether it is a cold or the flu, the physically fit individual will usually recover faster than the out-of-shape person.

In summary, we believe that every executive can benefit from a program of exercise, provided that a physician gives him or her the green light. This is true especially for those who have one or more of the cardiovascular risk factors, but it also applies to those with no detectable risks. Experience has taught us that if executives exercise regularly, they become much more adept at performing their usual daily activities at work and at home, and this includes sex. Sexual activity involves vigorous movement. The better the physical shape you are in, the more you will be able to engage in strenuous sexual activity without risking fatigue.

Seventy-eight-year-old Senator Strom Thurmond of South Carolina provides a good example of the effects of regular exercise. Thurmond is an avid runner. He has been taking a daily run of 2 to 4 miles for longer than he cares to remember. He married a woman in her thirties in 1968 when he was 65 years old. They now have four children.

Treating Stress through Exercise

Most executives face tremendous amounts of stress on the job, whether they are working conscientiously to advance up the corporate ladder or trying to stay on top. Stress can lead to a number of serious physical and emotional problems, including nervous disorders, ulcers, and cardiovascular complications. Exercise can help most executives relieve the stress involved in decision making, because exercise helps one avoid directing the stress and tension inwardly.

An executive cannot eliminate stress from life; the only way to do that would be to stop working. What an executive can do is reduce his or her reaction to stress. The best way to do that is to work off tension during regular vigorous physical workouts. EHE doctors do not recommend sedatives or tranquilizers for executives beset by everyday stresses; we recommend exercise. In Chapter 3 we will explain and recommend the exercises we believe are best for executives.

Well-conditioned patients seem to have an easier time tolerating disease.

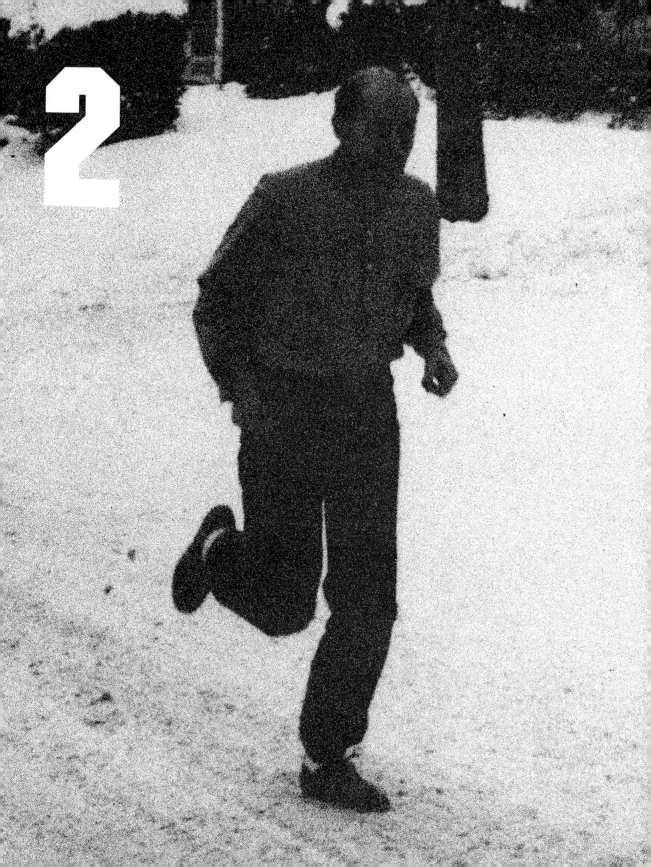

CHOOSING YOUR EXERCISE PROGRAM

A recent European visitor to the United States remarked that the first thing he noticed in the large cities he visited was "a lot of people running around in their underwear." He was talking about the ubiquitous urban jogger, of course, the most visible manifestation of a physical fitness explosion that began in the early 1970s in this country. By the end of the decade, opinion polls showed that for the first time more than half of all Americans aged 18 and over were participating in some form of daily physical exercise. Nearly 60 percent of the adults questioned in the 1978 Harris Poll, for example, said they took part in a regular exercise program that lasted $2\frac{1}{2}$ hours or more a week. About 15 percent said they exercised more than 5 hours a week. In comparison, only about 24 percent of those questioned in 1961 reported that they exercised regularly.

As the European visitor noted, the jogger/runner is the most visible symbol of today's exercise explosion. There are now tens of millions of regular joggers in every corner of the land, traversing the nation's roads, exploring its parks, and circling its athletic fields. Dozens of books have been published in the last decade on various facets of jogging and running, including the 1977 best-seller *The Complete Book of Running* by James Fixx. Jogging, however, is only one of many forms of exercise now being practiced regularly that offer the same physical and psychological benefits.

Aerobics, Stretching, and Strength Building

Jogging/running is classified as an aerobic exercise, or one that is maintained in a continuous, rhythmic manner. The aerobic exercises are named for the Greek word for *air* because they stimulate increases in oxygen-bearing blood flow, inducing the heart to work harder and thereby expanding the blood vessels.

Medical research strongly indicates that aerobic exercises—which include running/jogging, walking, swimming, bicycling, rope skipping, and cross-country skiing—develop and maintain cardiovascular fitness and body strength. Doctors believe that a regular exercise program that includes as its basis an aerobic program probably will aid in the preven-

JOGGING VERSUS RUNNING

What is the difference between jogging and running? Jogging seems to imply running at low speeds, whereas running seems to mean jogging at fast speeds. As for other differences, even the experts do not agree. Here is how some of them compare the two:

"Although some would argue the point, there is no particular speed at which jogging turns into running. If you feel that you're running, no matter how slow you're going, no one can say you're not. For purposes of the present discussion, therefore, it's all referred to as running, no matter what the speed."

James F. Fixx, *The Complete Book of Running*, 1977, p. xvii

"Jogging is a pace slower than seven minutes per mile. When you cover a mile in less than seven minutes you're running . . . a 'runner' is one who competes against others. A 'jogger' only competes against

herself. You can see, therefore, that a person may be a jogger one day and a runner the next."

Guidelines for Successful Jogging, American Running and Fitness Association (formerly the National Jogging Association), 1977.

"Jogging is once or twice around the block in your baggy high-school sweats. Running is when you measure time or distance and strive for goals."

Frank Shorter, Olympic gold medalist, quoted in *Business Week*, November 7, 1977.

"Jogging is the stage between walking and running. During walking one foot is always touching the ground, whereas in running both feet are clear of the ground for an extended period of time. Jogging is seen as the time when the body leaves the ground to become airborne for some period of stride. In other words, jogging is a slow, easy form of running. It starts for most people at 4.5 to 5.0 miles per hour. Just where jogging ends and running begins is not defined. It may be a psychological point where you decide you will move along to get where you want to go as fast as you can."

Alan J. Ryan, M.D., sports physician and editor of *The Physician and Sportsmedicine*, quoted in *The Cardiologists' Guide to Fitness and Health through Exercise*, 1979.

"Distinctions between running and jogging are not very helpful. Jogging is running, but it's generally thought to be running long, slow distances. Its goal is elevation of the pulse rate to a level that is consistent with your level of fitness, age and capability."

Bernard L. Gladieux, Jr., former managing editor of *Running & Fitness* (formerly *The Jogger*), an American Running and Fitness Association (formerly the National Jogging Association) publication, in a personal interview.

"Anything faster than a nine-minute mile I call running. Anything slower I call jogging."

Kenneth H. Cooper, M.D., *The Aerobics Way*, 1977.

tion of coronary disease and could prolong one's life. It is known for certain that aerobic exercises can help you lose weight and keep it off. Moreover, most people who continue an aerobic program for at least 6 months find that they look healthier and feel stronger and more confident.

Much of the credit for today's wide interest in aerobic exercise goes to former Air Force physician Kenneth H. Cooper. In the early 1960s, Cooper developed the theory of aerobics after conducting extensive tests to measure the effects of aerobic exercise on volunteers' cardiovascular systems and overall health. The term *aerobic exercise* began to be used popularly after the publication of Cooper's first book, *Aerobics*, in 1968. He has since published two expanded aerobics books: *The New Aerobics* (1970) and *The Aerobics Way* (1977).

Cooper's basic theory is that aerobic exercise increases the body's consumption of oxygen by increasing the strength and capacity of the vehicles for supply and delivery: the lungs and the heart. In so doing, aerobic exercises im-

> Aerobic exercises improve the overall condition of the body, make the heart work more efficiently, and probably build resistance to illness and disease.

prove the overall condition of the body, make the heart work more efficiently, and probably build resistance to illness and disease. Executive Health Examiners recommends that every executive incorporate one of the aerobic exercises into his or her regular exercise program. The aerobic programs we recommend will be spelled out in detail in Chapters 3 and 4.

Stretching Exercises

While aerobics should be the basis of a balanced exercise program, no such program is complete without the incorporation of a series of stretching exercises. These routines are designed to make the muscles more flexible and relaxed and to mitigate the effects of stress. They help extend and maintain the range of movement in specific joints and series of joints. All the major muscle groups should be stretched regularly. Many doctors recommend paying special attention to the lower back, which is particularly susceptible to soreness and pain. Joggers, runners, walkers, and cyclists should also pay close attention to the thigh and leg muscles. These muscles should be well stretched before one takes part in aerobic exercises. For more details on stretching exercises, see Chapter 5.

Strength-Building Exercises

The third component of a balanced exercise program consists of muscular strength exercises. Think back to the executive described in Chapter 1 whose exercise regimen consisted only of situps and pushups. These two strength-building exercises helped him build up his stomach, back, arm, and chest muscles, but the man's exercise program was incomplete since it did not include any aerobic or flexibility exercises. We consider the program incomplete because strength-building exercises have only the most minute effect on the cardiovascular system and do not help stretch or relax the muscles. A body builder with rippling muscles may look like the healthiest person in the world, but underneath the bulging muscles could be a rapidly aging cardiovascular system. It does little good to build up the muscles without simultaneously building up the cardiovascular system.

The two basic kinds of strength-building exercises are isometrics and isotonics. Both systems involve overloading the muscles so that they are forced to work increasingly harder to lift progressively heavier loads. In isometric exercises, the muscle pushes against an immovable object such as a wall. This forces the muscle to contract and eventually to build up strength. Isotonic strength building involves lifting weights or using the body's movements, as in situps and pushups. Both isometric and isotonic exercises, if done properly, can be valuable parts of a total exercise program. You will not be totally healthy without strength, but strong muscles alone do not mean that you are totally healthy.

Who Needs a Stress Test?

A New England advertising executive, after hearing about the three-part balanced exercise regimen recommended by Executive Health Examiners, was ready to go home and work out a self-prescribed program. "Well, I've got the basics," he said, "and I can't wait to start my program." We asked him to wait and listen to a few other things about exercise first. We told him that some people can easily and safely prescribe their own balanced exercise programs by choosing one of the aerobic exercises, one of the flexibility exercises, and one of the strength-building exercises. If they practice each exercise for a given amount of time for a certain number of days a week, they soon will reap the physiological and psychological benefits.

We also told this man that since he was 39 years old, there was at least one very important thing he needed to do before starting his exercise program: take a stress test. At Executive Health Examiners we do *not* automatically give every executive embarking on an exercise program a stress test, but we do advise every executive starting an exercise program who is over 35 years old to take one. According to the American Heart Association, as many as 10 percent of men over 35 with no overt symptoms have some form of hidden heart disease, whereas only about 1 percent of those under 35 with no symptoms do. A stress test can uncover hidden heart disease.

Executive Health Examiners follows the advice given by the American College of Sports Medicine in recommending what type of physical examination should be given before the start of an exercise program.

To summarize briefly, if you are under 35 and are physically active, you have little to worry about as you embark on an exercise program. But if you are physically inactive, regardless of your age, it's best to be prudent and have a physical examination before you begin exercising. The physical should include tests of your cardiovascular system and blood pressure and an examination of your muscles and joints. Your cholesterol and triglyceride levels should be determined, and you should be given a resting electrocardiograph (EKG) test.

The most important part of the physical examination is the exercise stress test, which we recommend for everyone over 35. The stress test is usually given on a stationary bicycle or a treadmill. The individual being tested pedals or jogs

According to the American Heart Association, 10 percent of men over 35 may have some form of hidden heart disease.

BEFORE YOU BEGIN AN EXERCISE PROGRAM

If You Are	*You Need To*
Any age, with no diseases, are physically active, and have no coronary heart disease risk factors or diseases	have only the barest amount of supervision. Consult a physician only when you are radically altering your exercise program.
Under 35, with no diseases, are physically inactive, and have no coronary risk factors or disease	consult a physician only if you have not had a medical evaluation during the previous year. Otherwise, you can work out your own physical fitness regimen with minimal risk.
Over 35, with no diseases, are physically inactive, and have no coronary heart disease risk factors or disease *or* Any age, with no diseases, are physically active or inactive, with coronary heart disease risk factors but no known disease	have a complete medical evaluation including a stress test administered by a certified technician
Any age, with known coronary heart disease *or* Any age, physically active or inactive, with known coronary heart disease but with no problems for 6 months or longer	get a careful evaluation of your specific medical problems and required medication and take a stress test with a physician in attendance.
Any age, with recent onset of coronary heart disease	same as above, plus get a thorough careful assessment of signs and symptoms and get an EKG and evaluation of required medication

SOURCE: Adapted from American College of Sports Medicine, *Guidelines for Graded Exercise Testing and Exercise Prescription*, 2d ed., (Philadelphia: Lea & Febiger, 1980), pp. 2–8.

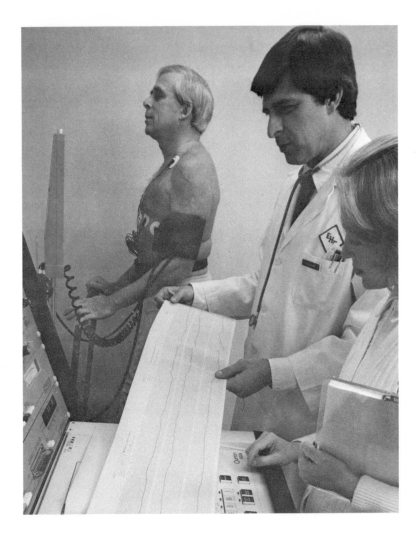

at increasing rates of speed until his or her ultimate capacity is reached. While this is going on, the following measurements are taken: pulse rate, electrocardiogram, blood pressure, and muscle fatigue. As the load is intensified, the body's responses are evaluated, and the stress test can pick up signs of previously hidden heart problems.

It should be pointed out that stress tests are not always accurate. On occasion a stress test will indicate that the patient has some sort of heart problem, but more extensive tests will show that there is nothing amiss. Conversely, a stress test sometimes will show that a patient has no heart irregularities when, in fact, they may exist. The medical terms for these two circumstances are false positives and false negatives, respectively. The stress test, then, is not perfect, but it is the best indicator doctors now have of how the body responds to exercise.

Executive Health Examiners uses the results of the stress test to prescribe an executive's individual exercise regimen. We believe that for the most part the test clearly and precisely measures the subject's fitness level, or the ability of the body to perform a certain amount of work. A stress test also serves as a good indicator of exercise and fitness progress.

For example, a 45-year-old marketing vice president took a stress test 3 years ago, and the results showed a very low capacity. He began an exercise program after the first stress test, and in each of his two annual stress test checkups since then he has shown marked improvement in several fitness categories. His cholesterol and blood pressure levels went down each year; his heartbeat at rest lowered several beats each year. The last time he came in for a physical, he told us that whenever he needs motivation to stick with his exercises, he reminds himself how long it will be before he

BASICS OF THE EHE EXERCISE REGIMEN

- *Type:* One aerobic, one strength-building, and one flexibility exercise. All three may be done in one session

- *Frequency:* Three sessions at the minimum, but preferably five sessions per week for all three types. Do not let more than 2 days go by between sessions.

- *Duration:* For aerobic exercise: 20 to 30 minutes per session. For stretching exercises: 10 to 15 minutes per session. For strength-building exercises: 10 to 15 minutes per session.

These may be combined into one 40 to 60-minute session

- *Intensity:* This is a subjective component, and for most persons it requires an individualized prescription based on the results of a physical examination. For those over 35, the physical should include a stress test. Remember the one absolute: Begin slowly and gradually. As Kenneth Cooper, author of *Aerobics*, says: "More speed or intensity too soon is like taking a whole bottle of medicine instead of just the recommended dosage —an invitation to trouble. . . ."

gets on the treadmill again. We have learned from his experience, and from many other similar cases, that the stress test not only is an indicator of progress but also can be a good motivator.

The Exercise Regimen: Type, Frequency, Duration, and Intensity

The four basic components of the EHE exercise regimen are the type, frequency, duration, and intensity of the exercises chosen for the program.

Type As we have seen, there are three basic types of exercise in the balanced program: aerobic, stretching, and strength building. We will review, analyze, and suggest the specific types of exercises in these areas in later chapters, but among the aerobic exercises, Executive Health Examiners recommends any one of the following: walking, jogging or running, bicycling (indoors on a stationary machine or outdoors on a regular bike), swimming, and rope skipping. There are other aerobic exercises, including skating, rowing, cross-country skiing, and strenuous games such as basketball, but we do not recommend them. Our experience working with hundreds of executives in exercise programs has shown that walking, running, cycling, swimming, and rope skipping are particularly suited to the executive lifestyle.

Another factor we stress: Once you have chosen an aerobic exercise, stick with it. Do not switch from cycling one week to swimming the next and jogging the next and so on. Think about what you like, what you do not like, and what you do well. Then look into the different aerobic exercises and choose one. If you choose an aerobic exercise you cannot abide by, leave it and go on to another, but choose the next one carefully so that you can stick with it, become proficient at it, and receive the maximum benefit from it.

For the stretching component of your balanced exercise program you may use any type of flexibility movements that are performed slowly and aid you in gradually progressing to a greater range of motion. You may choose several yoga stretching positions, for example, making sure that you take the time to stretch all the large muscle groups of the body.

Once you have chosen an aerobic exercise, stick with it.

We recommend a number of different types of muscular strength-building exercises. You can practice isometric exercises, using immovable objects. These require extremely strenuous but very brief expenditures of strength. You also can lift weights in the isotonic method. You can buy a chinup bar and work out on it, or you can use the old stand-bys, pushups and situps. The thing to keep in mind here is to work on building up strength equally in the arms, back, and legs.

Frequency There can be no real benefit in an exercise program if it is not performed regularly. We therefore recommend that you exercise at least three times a week and that you do not allow more than 2 days to go by between sessions. For the working executive a good schedule would be Monday, Wednesday, and Friday or Tuesday, Thursday, and Saturday, but you can gain even more from exercising five times a week. A good habit to get into is to exercise each weekday at a set time, either before or after work or during the lunch hour. The minimum of three sessions and the maximum of five hold true for all three components of the exercise program. It also is a good idea to do all three during the same session.

Duration This brings us to the all-important question of time. We will deal with suggestions on how to fit the exercise regimen into the busy executive's schedule later in this chapter, but for now let us discuss how much time you will need. In order to gain the minimum benefit from an aerobic program, you need to spend at least 20 minutes with your heart working at about three-quarters of its maximum capacity, in the so-called target zone. You should not reach this plateau immediately after you start exercising, nor should you stop exercising immediately after you have been at this plateau for 20 minutes. You need both a warmup period and a cooling-down period.

The good news for time-conscious executives is that you can use warmup and cooling-down time to do your stretching and strength-building exercises. If you spend 10 to 15 minutes warming up with stretches and some situps, push-ups, and other calisthenics and another 10 to 15 minutes cooling down with more stretching, your total daily exercise period should last about 45 to 60 minutes, or nearly an hour a session. This is the absolute minimum, and it bears repeating. The minimal exercise session should consist of about 10 to 15 minutes of stretching, 20 to 30 minutes of aerobic activity, and 10 to 15 minutes of strength building. That amounts to a 40- to 60-minute session, and you should do at least three, and preferably five, of these sessions a week.

Intensity The intensity of an exercise program is the most subjective and personal component. Just how far you should push yourself requires an individualized exercise prescription, preferably formulated after reviewing the results of a stress test. Remember, the most important rule for anyone starting an exercise program is to begin *slowly*. The temptation, of course, is to set high goals and try to attain them quickly. No one wants to admit that at age 41, for example, he or she no longer has the physical capacity to run cross-country races. This is very hard to explain to ex-athletes. Many executives we work with at Executive Health Examiners have in their younger days been active in organized sports. When they make the decision to try to get back into shape, they often forget that it has taken them many years, and sometimes decades, to put their bodies out of shape. The tendency is to try to get back to where they once were in a matter of days.

The minimal exercise session should consist of about 10 or 15 minutes of stretching, 20 to 30 minutes of aerobic activity, and 10 to 15 minutes of strength building.

Dr. Cooper says that the "cardinal rule" of aerobics is "safely, slowly and progressively," and that goes for the other parts of your exercise program as well. "More speed or intensity too soon," Cooper writes, "is like taking a whole bottle of medicine instead of just the recommended dosage —an invitation to trouble, in this case from tendons, muscles, joints and your heart."[1]

Time Constraints

"I know I should take part in an exercise program," a 36-year-old vice president of a publishing firm told an EHE doctor at a recent checkup. "But I just don't have the time." Not having the time is the number one answer executives give when asked why they do not exercise. We have found that there is no lack of interest in exercise among executives, but there is a lack of time, or at least a perceived lack. The publishing executive told us that she has to catch a 6:40 A.M. train to get to work in New York City. When she gets off the train, she has just enough time to hop aboard the subway that takes her to work. She usually is tied up nearly every day in business lunches and therefore cannot exercise during the day. When she gets home from work, it's time for dinner. "I sit down and eat, and then the evening is gone," she told us. "Where do I fit in exercise?"

We told this woman what we tell all executives with this complaint. Believe it or not, you can fit a complete, balanced exercise program into a busy executive schedule without sacrificing anything, either on the job or at home. We believe that you should not fit that hour of exercise into your schedule—you should instead fit your schedule around that hour of exercise.

Dr. Nora puts it this way: If your "schedule is already so full that there's no way you can fit another hour a day into it . . . then it becomes even more imperative that you do just that. Take an hour away from the hassle and invest it in saving your life. This hour absolutely must not be looked on as just another hour to add to your other conflicting de-

[1] Kenneth H. Cooper, *The Aerobics Way* (1977), p. 66.

mands. You must not think of it that way or approach it that way. This hour is yours. It's for you and your life and your well-being: It's first priority. There's nothing you have to do that's more important."[2]

Here is how we solved the publishing executive's time dilemma. When we explained how important we believed that hour to be, she sat down with us, and we reexamined her daily schedule. Before long we were able to help her find the time for an exercise regimen. She followed our suggestion and was able to fulfill the aerobic component of her exercise program easily. She had been taking the subway from the train station in the city to her office a mile and a half away. Instead of riding the subway, she began walking that distance at a brisk enough pace—about 5 miles an hour—to get aerobic benefits. She even made it to work on time.

The publishing executive also discovered another beneficial side effect of her morning walk. When she finished the brisk 15-minute walk, she was not dripping with sweat or exhausted. In fact, she was ready for the morning's work, feeling freshly invigorated and mentally alert. She soon stopped eating heavy breakfasts before leaving for work, because they did not sit well during her morning walk. Instead, she ate a light breakfast and was not at all hungry when she got to the office. She used to eat an occasional doughnut during the morning coffee break. After she began the walking routine, she only wanted something lighter and soon switched to fruit juice.

The Right Time to Exercise

As this example illustrates, with proper motivation a way can be found to carve out an exercise routine that does not disrupt a regimented, time-filled daily work routine. One way to find that time is to look at three periods during the day: in the morning before work, in the evening after work, and in the afternoon during lunch hour. The way for an executive to find out which of these periods is best is to exam-

---

[2] James Jackson Nora, *The Whole Heart Book* (New York: Holt, Rinehart and Winston, 1980), p. 154.

Believe it or not, you *can* fit a complete, balanced exercise program into a busy schedule without sacrificing anything.

ine his or her schedule. If, for instance, your one-way commute between home and the office is between 1.5 and 4 miles, think about getting your aerobic exercise by either walking or jogging to work. You may eventually also want to walk or jog home as well. You do not have to do this every day of the week—3 days is sufficient—but once you get in the habit, you may discover you enjoy walking or jogging to work, and you may want to do it each weekday, except perhaps for days when there is particularly inclement weather.

If you live 3 to 10 miles from the office, you might consider riding a bicycle to and from work. You can easily get aerobic benefits in this manner. Or, like the publishing executive, you can take public transportation part of the way to work and walk briskly for the last 1.5 to 2 miles. Another option is to drive your car within a few miles of where you work, carrying your bicycle on a rack. You can then park the car and ride the bike the last 3 to 10 miles. A 37-year-old EHE client who lives 25 miles from work has used this method for 6 years. He says the commute takes only 10 minutes longer than normal using the car-bike method, and he avoids the nerve-wracking (and stress-building) experience of fighting city rush-hour traffic, not to mention rates for a parking space in the city.

If for some reason you cannot work your exercise routine into your daily commute, try setting aside three to five lunch hours a week for exercise. Many companies have installed gymnasiums in their office complexes. If your office does not have one, you have other options. You can join the many other lunch-hour joggers out in the streets and parks, or you can take a brisk 30 to 45-minute walk and window-shop your way to better health. You also can go to a health club, gym, or yoga class during lunch.

Whatever time period you choose, experiment to see what suits your schedule. If you cannot fit in an exercise regimen in the morning, try the evening hours after you get home from work, or try getting up a bit earlier. You might just stumble into a perfect time, but you will never know until you experiment and try.

There are other times of the day during which you can exercise. We have learned from many of our patients that it is possible to work all the exercises into a daily executive schedule. Some of them eschew elevators during the day at work; instead they walk briskly up and down stairwells. Just bolting up a staircase for a few seconds does not provide aerobic benefit; this is classified as an anaerobic exercise, or one that provides no cardiovascular benefit. But there are physiologic benefits, including helping the leg muscles become stronger, to be gained by moving out from behind your desk and hitting the stairs. Above all, the activity keeps you from stagnating, both mentally and physically, in your sedentary job.

Two EHE doctors have devised a walking routine which they undertake while waiting for the commuter train on the way home from the office each evening. During the wait, which sometimes lasts up to 30 minutes, they walk briskly from one end of the platform to the other. Fifteen minutes of walking provides them with aerobic exercise for the day. A number of EHE patients make it a practice to walk to all their appointments in the city during working days. Some executives get off the bus several stops before work and walk rapidly for the last mile or two to the office.

There are many stretching and isometric exercises you can do while driving to work or while sitting as a passenger in a car, train, or airplane. In fact, there is a book, *Autocize*,

There are many exercises you can do while driving to work or while sitting in a car, train, or airplane.

by Jay David, that explains exactly how to do these sorts of exercises. David suggests one stretching program for men and women who spend at least a half hour a day in a car. It's a 4-day program with each day set aside to exercise a different muscle group. One day you concentrate on the head and neck, the next day on the arms, then the waist and buttocks, and finally the legs and feet. The exercises range from full body stretching while standing outside the car before you begin to drive and isometrics using the car's fenders, to neck stretches and leg raises while you are driving.

Exercising on a Business Trip

For the executive on a business trip, there are many chances to exercise. Some hotels offer out-of-town guest maps of the surrounding area's best running paths, and some have swimming pools and gyms. If possible, it's a good idea to stay at a hotel that caters to executives with regular exercise schedules. James Fixx suggests that the best time to exercise while out of town often is about an hour before dinner:

> Meetings tend to break up about five o'clock, and dinner is commonly scheduled for seven. Some people go to their rooms for a bath and a rest; others gather for a drink or two. That's the time to go running [or do any other aerobic exercise]. The chances are that you won't even be missed but if your disappearance will be noticed and commented upon, don't hesitate to announce, 'Well, time for a little jog.' People will admire you for it.[3]

[3] James Fixx, *The Complete Book of Running* (New York: Random House, 1977), pp. 129—130.

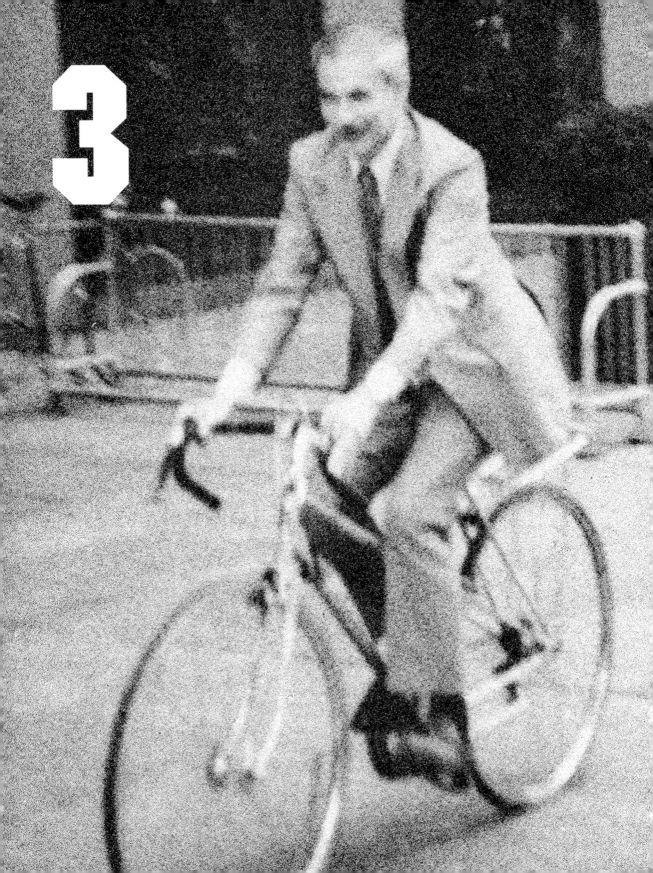

AEROBICS: THE KEY TO THE EXECUTIVE FITNESS REGIMEN

When biologists talk about *aerobes*, they are referring to organisms that can live only in the presence of oxygen. When physicians refer to *aerobics*, they are talking about exercises that impel the human body to use oxygen more efficiently. Aerobic exercises increase the flow of blood to the heart, and this blood supplies life-giving oxygen to all of the body's muscles and organs. The body's ability to deliver oxygen to the heart and skeletal muscles is the prime determinant of physical fitness. The more efficiently oxygen is supplied to the heart and muscles, the better the level of physical fitness, because an efficient flow of oxygen allows a person to exercise vigorously without undue fatigue.

The way to determine the efficiency of your flow of oxygen is to notice your condition after vigorous activity such as running. If running for 10 minutes causes you to gasp for breath, your cardiovascular system is not pumping blood efficiently. As your heart pounds and you try to catch your breath, your lungs are trying desperately to pump more oxygen-bearing blood throughout your body, and they are failing.

You may have noticed that long-distance runners do not gasp for breath after a race. This is because their cardiovascular systems are operating at peak efficiency, delivering large volumes of blood throughout their bodies quickly as they call on their muscles to perform.

Aerobic exercises are the key to the EHE executive fitness regimen because they improve the body's blood, lung, and heart functions by facilitating delivery of oxygen to these tissues. In addition, aerobic exercises provide beneficial side effects that you will feel every hour of every day. If you practice an aerobic exercise routine faithfully for several months, you will begin to notice that you are feeling less tired throughout the day; your cardiovascular system will be working, like the long-distance runner's, at peak efficiency. You may not be able to run a mile in under 4 minutes, but at 4 P.M. on a hectic Friday you should have sufficient reserve energy to be mentally alert and physically strong enough to perform any task at hand.

Dr. Cooper describes the consequences for the sedentary individual who does not undertake an aerobic program. Such an individual will more than likely have to face the "symptoms of inactivity," Cooper writes, such as "yawning at your desk, that drowsy feeling all day, falling asleep after a heavy meal, fatigue from even mild exertions like climbing stairs, running for a bus, mowing the lawn or shoveling snow." Cooper warns that a sedentary executive not getting aerobic exercise "can become a social cripple, 'too tired' to play with the kids, 'too tired' to go out to dinner with your wife, 'too tired' to do anything except sit at your desk or watch television, and maybe you're even getting tired doing that."[1]

Your Pulse, Pulse Taking, and the Target Zone

The main object of aerobic exercise is to increase the heartbeat to a level at which large amounts of oxygenated blood are pumped throughout the body. To reach that level, you must get your heart beating at between 70 and 85 percent of its maximal attainable rate. This level is called the *target zone.* Anything lower than that does not stimulate the heart

[1] Kenneth H. Cooper, *Aerobics*, p. 27.

Aerobic exercises are the key to the EHE fitness regimen because they improve the body's blood, lung, and heart functions.

enough. Anything higher, and you may hit a danger point that can overstress the heart. The best way to determine your own target zone is to locate your age on the accompanying chart. Your target zone is the shaded area that indicates the heart rate in beats per minute (BPM) that is between 70 and 85 percent of your age group's maximal heart rate.

The way to find out if you are in the target zone (and getting maximal aerobic benefit from your exercise) is to check your pulse during and after an exercise period. As a measure of the heartbeat, the pulse is 98 percent accurate. There are eleven pulse points in the body. To take your own pulse, the best point to use is a carotid artery located on either side of the throat. You can feel your pulse by placing your thumb on your chin and your four fingers on the side of your neck and gently pressing into the throat. Use a watch while you count the number of beats for 10 seconds and then multiply that number by 6 to determine your pulse rate.

Beginners should check the pulse several times during the exercise period. Take the first pulse after your warmup. At this point, before you begin aerobic activity, your pulse should be below the target zone. Then, 3 to 5 minutes into your aerobic activity, take the pulse again to make sure you have reached the lower limits of your target zone. (If you are below the target zone, step on it; you need to increase your intensity. If you are over the target zone and into the danger zone, *slow down.*) Finally, take your pulse immediately upon finishing aerobic exercise. Waiting a few seconds will not give an accurate measure, because the heartbeat decreases rapidly when you stop exercising. After a few months of steady aerobic activity, you will not need to check your pulse often. After 6 months, you will know your body's reaction well enough to tell intuitively when you are in the target zone.

Achieving the Target Zone

Your warmup period should serve as a gradual transition from inactivity to aerobic activity. Take it easy for the first few minutes and then gradually increase the intensity of your stretching and calisthenics. When you begin aerobic activity, do not try to get your heart into the target zone immediately. This is akin to revving up the engine of a sports car and shifting directly from first to fifth gear; the car is not designed to be used in this fashion. If you do not go through all five gears in sequence, you can wreck the engine. The same dangers are present when you push your body too strenuously in too short a period of time. The aim is to stay in the target zone for at least 20 minutes per aerobic session. It's perfectly all right to be under the target zone for 5 minutes or so as you begin doing aerobic exercises.

If you stay within the target zone, you will soon be rewarded. The prime benefit of sustained aerobic exercise is the improvement of cardiovascular capacity, or what is called the training effect. When this happens, you will be able to run, walk, cycle, swim, or skip rope for longer periods of time without feeling overly tired. This is due to the physiological changes that occur in the heart after a few weeks of aerobic training. In essence, you are building up your heart muscle and making your heart stronger and more efficient. A strong heart pumps an increased volume of blood with each beat, which allows oxygen to be transported more rapidly throughout the entire body. With this enhanced circula-

Beginners should check their pulse several times during the exercise period.

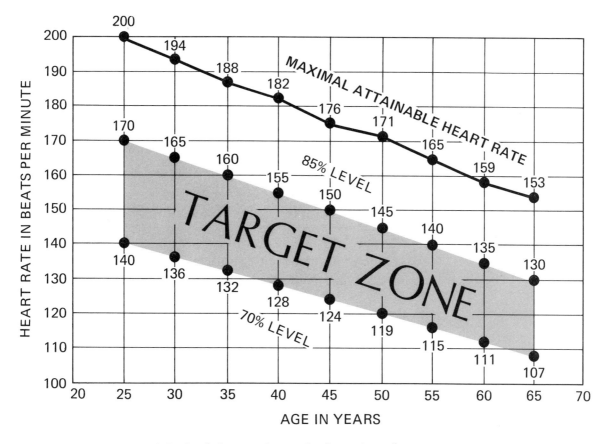

tion comes a toning of the body's muscles and a lowering of the blood pressure.

Then comes what is perhaps the most dramatic evidence that your cardiovascular system is in good shape. Your resting heartbeat decreases. Of course, it will not go as low as Frank Shorter's. The 1972 Olympic marathon champion has a resting heartbeat of 34 beats per minute. But then again, he runs 17 miles a day when he is in training. With continued aerobic exercising, your resting heartbeat can drop from the average 70 to 80 per minute to 55 to 65 after a year of aerobic training. When your resting heartbeat lowers, your heart beats thousands of times fewer each day. Although it has not been proved that humans are built with a finite number of heartbeats, it makes sense that the fewer times your heart beats each day, the less you are demanding of that vital organ.

What type of aerobic exercise is best for you?

Choosing an Aerobic Program

A common question among executives about to embark on an exercise program is, What type of aerobic exercise is best for me? There are at least twenty different aerobic exercises to choose from, including walking, jogging/running, cycling, swimming, cross-country skiing, roller skating/ice skating, rope jumping, running in place, chair stepping, stationary bicycling, rowing machine, treadmill, jumping jacks, dancing, handball/squash, soccer, basketball, sculling/canoeing, and just about any other activity you can imagine that stimulates the heart and lungs for 20 to 30 minutes so that the heart rate is elevated to 70 to 85 percent of maximum capacity. See the accompanying box for an illustration of these aerobic exercises.

Executive Health Examiners does not recommend the majority of these exercises for executives for two basic reasons. They may be impractical for most executives to practice on a regular, year-round basis, or they may not be efficient in terms of energy expended per minute. Only five aerobic exercises meet these and other EHE criteria: walking, running/jogging, swimming, cycling (indoors or outdoors), and rope skipping. These five aerobic regimens also require very little special equipment and can easily be worked into a crowded daily schedule.

These five exercises also offer two additional benefits. Along with cross-country skiing, they cause the body to expend a level of energy that will allow you to reach the target zone and stay within its limits comfortably and without undue strain. These exercises, moreover, are easily suited to precise, uncomplicated measurement of performance, allowing you to keep track of your progress in terms of miles (or laps) covered per session. It's much more difficult to keep track of week-to-week improvement in programs which do not lend themselves to precise measurement, such as aerobic dancing or canoeing.

Choosing Your Personal Exercise Regimen

Now that we have narrowed the list to five exercises, how do you choose among them? The most important thing—really the only important thing, since they all provide the same benefits—is making sure that the exercise you choose suits you. One client of Executive Health Examiners, the president of a New York City accounting firm, provides an example of what can happen if you choose an exercise that does not suit you.

Our client took up jogging after we pointed out the benefits of aerobic exercise. He told us that he had never liked running, but he was willing to give it a try because he knew that it would help him. He later told us he had hated every minute of every run he took during the 6 months he stuck with the program. "The only thing I think about when I'm running is how soon it will be before I stop," he said. Obviously, this man was not suited for running, and it took a bit of persuading before he was ready to try another aerobic routine. He was pleasantly surprised to learn that he actually enjoyed his second aerobic choice, bicycling, and he has continued to cycle three times a week.

Another way to choose an aerobic exercise is to determine which one suits your physical capacities. If you have especially strong legs, try running or cycling. If you are an accomplished recreational swimmer, look no further than

Basketball	Rope skipping*	**AEROBIC**
Chair stepping	Rowing machine	**EXERCISING**
Cycling*	Running in place	**ROUTINES**
Cross-country skiing	Sculling/canoeing	
Dancing	Soccer	
Handball/squash	Stationary bicycling*	
Jogging/running*	Swimming*	
Jumping jacks	Walking*	
Roller skating/ice skating		

* Recomended by Executive Health
Examiners for executives.

swimming. If you have always been well coordinated and quick on your feet, try rope skipping. If you are overweight, try walking. Walking is the least strenuous of the recommended aerobic exercises and is especially suited to the sedentary executive who has been inactive for many years. Many executives start their aerobic programs with walking and then go on to running or cycling after a few months. Many others find that they enjoy walking and stay with it.

Exercises We Do Not Recommend

Now for the aerobic exercises we do not recommend. Bear in mind that all the aerobic activities we have listed provide aerobic conditioning. Executive Health Examiners has found, though, that these exercises can present many problems for most executives. Nevertheless, if you find that one of them fits well into your schedule without unduly complicating your life and that you enjoy taking part in it, go ahead and make it your regular exercise program.

Here are some of the exercises we regard as causing problems: cross-country skiing, roller and ice skating, sculling, canoeing, dancing, and using a rowing machine. Exercises such as these can have drawbacks because they require an investment in too much equipment and usually also require ready access to facilities such as health clubs or special classes that are not available everywhere. Contrast this with running and walking. These exercises require only one piece of special equipment—a good pair of running shoes—and you can run or walk just about anywhere. Cycling, of course, does entail buying a sturdy indoor stationary bicycle or a decent ten-speed bike, but we feel that the benefits of cycling—especially the fact that it brings the heart to the target zone quickly—far outweigh the investment in equipment.

The same thing is true for swimming. An aerobic swimming program requires ready access to a swimming pool with lanes set up for exercising. For some executives finding such a pool might be as complicated as renting a canoe, making arrangements to store it in a boathouse, and paddling down a river on a 3-day-a-week basis. But if there is a

Running and walking require only one item of equipment: a good pair of running shoes.

swimming pool near where you work or live—and for most executives who live in or near a metropolitan area this should be no problem—we recommend swimming over exercises that require the use of outside facilities.

We do not recommend basketball, squash, or handball for most executives, especially those who have been inactive for many years. These sports are simply too strenuous for the average executive starting an aerobic program. In addition to that, they are competitive, and one of the objectives of the exercise prescription for executives is to provide a chance to escape from the competitive lifestyle of the office. Exercise is meant to help you relax, and a competitive sport often has the opposite effect. We therefore strongly suggest that only executives in top cardiovascular shape take up basketball, squash, and handball for aerobic exercise.

The Problem of Boredom

The final group of aerobic exercises we do not recommend includes chair stepping, running in place, and jumping jacks. They are on our reject list for one basic reason: they can easily become exceedingly boring. All aerobic exercises are repetitive, but at least the scenery changes when you run, walk, or cycle outdoors, and the indoor rope-skipping routine requires dexterity and coordination. Chair stepping, running in place, and jumping jacks, however, are so monotonously repetitive that there is a very real possibility you will be so bored after a few weeks that you will quit exercising and never go back to it.

But, you might object, Executive Health Examiners recommends the exercise bicycle. What could be more boring than sitting on an indoor stationary bike and staring at a wall for 20 minutes at a time three days a week? Several of our clients have provided a solution to that problem. One 32-year-old publishing executive told us she moved her exercise cycle in front of the television soon after she took up the exercise. She gets on the cycle early in the morning and watches the network news while pedaling her way to cardiovascular health.

Another EHE client, a 45-year-old vice president of an investment firm, came to us soon after his father died of a heart attack. The man was not athletic and disliked exercising, but he decided that because of a family history of heart disease, he needed to improve his cardiovascular condition. When we listed the five recommended aerobic exercises, he chose the exercise bicycle but soon became bored. We suggested that he try listening to the radio or watching television while he cycled, but neither solution suited him.

He soon came up with his own unique answer. He bought a cassette recorder equipped with lightweight headphones. Once a week he rents a prerecorded tape of a book and "reads" the book as he exercises. "I can't tell you how happy I am now," he said during a recent checkup. "I'm getting back to reading all the books I never had the chance to get to. And when I'm 'reading,' I barely think about the fact that I'm exercising. I now ride the bike for 3 to 4 hours a week."

The EHE Criteria for Choosing an Exercise Program

To sum up what is involved in choosing one of the five aerobic programs we recommend, here are the criteria once again:

First and most important, choose an exercise that suits you. Make sure that you enjoy taking part in it and that your body is suited to it. You may have played basketball on the college team and loved the sport, but if you have not played in 5 years, try walking or cycling for aerobic exercise. After you have built up your cardiovascular system, you can take up basketball again. Or if you have some type of leg injury, try swimming, a sport which puts no strain on the legs.

Second, choose an exercise that you can do without inconveniencing yourself unduly. If the only facility that has a treadmill or rowing machine is located an hour's drive from your house, it just does not pay to make that trip three times a week, especially when you can put on a pair of track shoes and run out the front door to get the same benefits. Obviously, if you live in New Orleans, you will not choose cross-country skiing; and if you live in Minneapolis, you will not choose sculling. Even if you live in a temperate climate, you may want to choose a program that can be done indoors so that you can avoid losing exercise time as a result of inclement weather.

Third, choose an exercise that can bring your heart to the target zone quickly. Each of the five recommended exercises fits this criterion. Cross-country skiing, basketball, squash, and handball also meet this requirement, but we rule them out for most executives for the reasons that were noted above.

Fourth, choose an exercise such as running, walking, swimming, cycling, or rope skipping in which you can measure your progress easily and precisely.

Golf and Tennis

A large number of executives play golf or tennis, and we are often asked whether these sports are good "exercises." The answer usually disappoints the golfers and does not exactly cheer the tennis players.

Golf provides no aerobic benefit and is not much use as a strength-building exercise. The only physiological benefit it

---

Golf provides no aerobic benefit and is not much use as a strength-building exercise.

Tennis players may not meet their need for exercise on the court.

gives is flexibility for the leg, arm, and chest muscles. But the golfer's routine of walking (if you are not riding a motorized cart), stopping, and hitting a ball does little to improve cardiovascular conditioning. However, there is an offbeat way to get aerobic benefit out of golfing. Lenore R. Zohman, M.D., and her colleagues describe it in their book *The Cardiologists' Guide to Fitness and Health through Exercise:*

> It's possible for a golfer to run in place between shots, run to and from the course or jog alongside the golf cart. However, the combination of golf shoes (not designed for running), loss of concentration on the golf game itself and the reaction of other players tends to make the prospect of such activity rather questionable.[2]

Executive Health Examiners recommends that if golf helps you relax, go out and play a round or two each week. But you still will have to take up a three-part exercise regimen of stretching, strength building, and aerobics in addition to your golf game.

The disappointing news for tennis players is that you may not be able to meet your exercise needs on the court. Tennis is a strenuous sport, and many executives who play it feel that it keeps them in good shape. As one corporate vice president who plays tennis twice a week told us, "I don't think I need anything else for exercise. I run around a lot on the court, my strokes make my arm and chest muscles work, and I work up a good sweat. It's great exercise."

When you look more closely at the body's physiological response to tennis, you can see that tennis is not an ideal aerobic exercise. Tennis, like volleyball, racketball, handball, and badminton, is a sport that consists of bursts of energy

[2] Lenore R. Zohman, Albert A. Kattus, and Donald G. Softness, *The Cardiologists Guide to Fitness and Health through Exercise* (New York: Simon and Schuster, 1979).

interspersed with brief rest periods. This takes away much of the aerobic benefit of the game, even though the heartbeat may be in the target zone for 20 to 30 minutes in the course of an hour on the court. The brief rest periods between serves, games, and sets negate much of the aerobic benefit. Dr. Cooper explains it this way: "You dash about the court chasing the ball, and the heart rate goes up to 150 or more. A point is scored and the action stops. The heart rate comes down to 120 or less. After a few games like this, the average heart rate is less than the 150 produced by non-stop aerobics."[3]

This is why Executive Health Examiners recommends to our clients who want to play tennis, and play it safely, that they get in shape first by practicing a fitness regimen. Tennis should not be the basis for fitness programing. We classify it as a beneficial side effect of a good overall exercise program. If you want to play tennis, you should not go out and play a vigorous singles game three times a week. You should work up to it gradually by building up your cardiovascular fitness through a balanced exercise regimen that stresses aerobics. You can improve your tennis through a half hour a day of other exercises. That way, when you do play tennis, you will be in better shape, be in better control, and play a more effective game.

Scientific evidence that tennis and golf do not provide high cardiovascular fitness was given in 1978 by Rudolph H. Dressendorfer of the Department of Physical Education at the University of California, Davis. Dressendorfer, a certified American College of Sports Medicine program director, undertook a study at the John A. Burns School of Medicine at the University of Hawaii to measure the cardiovascular fitness of a group of healthy men, 25 to 38 years old, whose major source of exercise was 3 to 6 hours a week of skin diving, golf, surfing, or tennis. The three golfers tested played two or three rounds (thirty-six to forty-five holes) a week and did not use motorized carts on the course; they walked. The two tennis players in the study played one or two sets of singles three times a week. All had been active for 2 years at their sports.

[3] Kenneth H. Cooper, *Aerobics*, p. 41.

Dressendorfer found that golf and tennis "appeared to be no more effective in developing satisfactory cardio-respiratory fitness than the normal physical activity of men entering an adult fitness program." Dressendorfer also tested these same men after they began a 3-day-a-week aerobic jogging program. After 3 months, all showed marked improvement in cardiovascular conditioning and aerobic capacity. Those who stayed in the jogging program an additional 3 months showed even more improvement.

"Our results indicate that these men had not attained high cardiorespiratory fitness through their recreational sports," Dressendorfer concluded, "and that jogging stimulated noteworthy improvement in oxygen consumption without significant changes in body weight or percentage of body fat."[4]

[4] Rudolph H. Dressendorfer, "Endurance Training of Recreationally Active Men," *The Physician and Sportsmedicine*, November 1978, pp. 123–131.

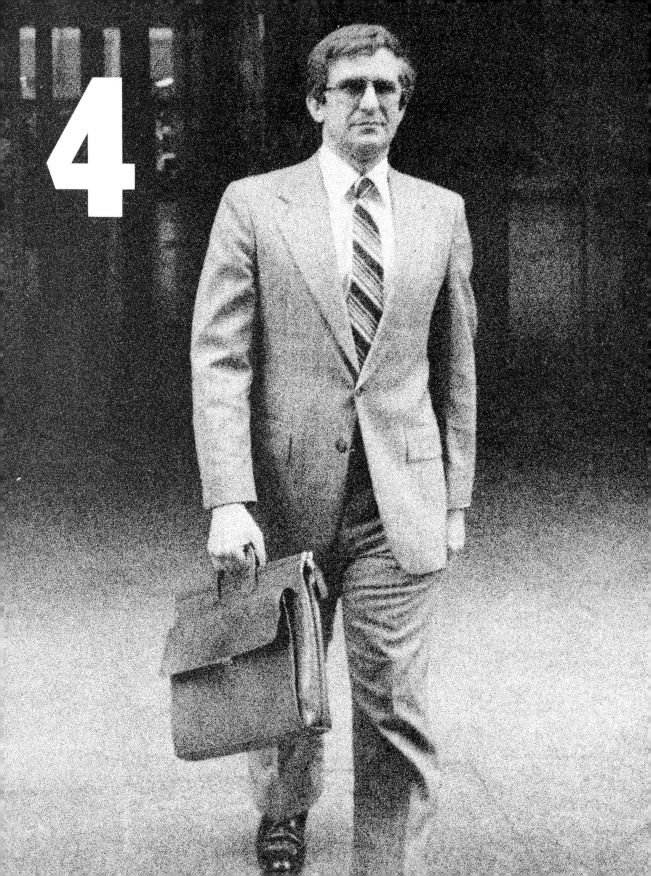

4

THE BEST AEROBIC EXERCISES FOR EXECUTIVES

As we pointed out in Chapter 3, five aerobic exercises—walking, running, cycling, swimming, and rope skipping—are especially suited for executives. In this chapter we will discuss the pluses and minuses of each of these exercises to help you decide which one is best for you. We will also tell you how to get started and how to fine-tune your aerobic routines as you make progress.

Each of these five exercises provides the same cardiovascular conditioning. The best way to choose the right exercise for yourself is to find one that suits you physically, that you enjoy taking part in, and that fits easily into your everyday schedule.

As we recommended in Chapter 2, you should take part in your aerobic exercise at least three but preferably five times a week. Each of these 20- to 30-minute aerobic sessions should be preceded by a 10- to 15-minute warmup consisting of a combination of stretching and calisthenics. After completing your aerobic routine, you should cool down with another 10- to 15-minute period of light stretching and more calisthenics.

As for the intensity with which you should exercise, remember that the object in aerobics is to bring your heartbeat to the target zone—between 70 and 85 percent of its maximal capacity. The only way to find out how much effort

The object in aerobics is to bring your heartbeat to the target zone—between 75 and 80 percent of its maximum capacity.

you need to expend to reach the target zone is to check your pulse frequently while doing aerobic exercises. If your heartbeat is below the target zone but you are too tired to work harder, do not push yourself. When you are exhausted, stop immediately. However, you should return to your exercise the next day. Within a few weeks, you will gradually build up your cardiovascular strength and be able to get to the target zone without straining.

If your heartbeat goes above the target zone, your body is telling you to slow down. You should lower the intensity with which you walk, run, swim, cycle, or skip rope and keep checking your pulse to see whether you are within the target zone.

The EHE aerobic exercise prescription is basically very simple. The primary objective is to keep your heartbeat in the target zone for 20 to 30 minutes three to five times a week. As you stay with the aerobic program, your cardiovascular fitness will improve and you will need to make adjustments to keep your heartbeat in the target zone for the required length of time.

It's a good idea to keep a written record of your aerobic activity. Devise a chart to keep track of the distance (or time) you spend exercising each day, along with your exercise pulse. Remember to progress gradually. Overstraining invites the risk of premanent injury.

Walking

Walking is by far the easiest and least complicated aerobic exercise. You do not have to learn how to walk, of course, and all you need in the way of equipment is a good pair of shoes.

We recommend walking either as a continuing aerobic exercise or as a transitional exercise before you move on to running or cycling. The basic walking rules are the same as those for all aerobic training.

* *After a 10 to 15 minute warmup, start walking slowly.*

* *Make sure you spend 20 to 30 minutes with your heartbeat in the target zone.*

* *Spend another 10 to 15 minutes cooling down.*

We recommend walking for executives of all ages and in all stages of physical condition, but several types of executives are especially good candidates for walking programs. Since walking, unlike running and cycling, presents few problems to people with leg injuries, we recommend it for those who are prone to shin splints or heel, ankle, knee, or other running-induced leg problems. We also recommend walking for executives 55 years of age or older for the same reason. Walking will not present a problem to older executives' more vulnerable hips, ankles, and other lower-body joints.

Executive Health Examiners recommends walking for overweight executives mainly because walking is the least strenuous aerobic exercise. We often recommend walking for executives who have arthritis. Some arthritis sufferers have found that walking helps the symptoms of the disease and also improves muscular flexibility. Some emphysema patients have also been helped by walking routines, and, of course, walking is now *de rigueur* for recuperating heart patients. Cardiologists have found that walking is the perfect exercise to stimulate the flow of blood throughout the body without putting undue strain on a heart patient's recovering cardiovascular system.

In short, walking is best for many sedentary executives because it requires a minimal level of exertion yet still provides aerobic benefits. As Charles T. Kuntzleman put it, there is "one fact that makes walking best of all for many people: the only exercise that does you any good is the exercise you do; and walking is very easy. It is less demanding than other aerobic exercises like swimming and running. If you're in reasonably good health—free of chest pain, dizziness, and high blood pressure—and if you use good judgment, you shouldn't have any problems."[1]

If you cannot believe that such an "easy" routine can actually improve cardiovascular conditioning, consider the results of a recent medical experiment in Israel. A series of tests conducted by doctors at the Heller Institute of Medical Research at Tel Aviv University Medical School measured the aerobic capacity of forty-four men aged 18 to 23. These young men walked about 3 miles per hour for 30 minutes a day, five days a week, carrying backpacks that weighed from 3 to 6 kilograms. Thirty-two men stayed with this program for 3 weeks; twelve stayed with it for 4 weeks. The doctors found that it is "possible to improve substantially aerobic physical fitness in three weeks by walking daily with a light backpack load." They also found that the walking regimen was "most useful for people who have low initial aerobic work." They recommended walking "as a gradual and safe method for improving physical fitness, mainly for people who have a low initial work capacity. Walking can easily be adapted as a way of life: everyone can use a briefcase or shopping bag instead of a backpack load."[2]

The Optimum Walking Pace

Executive Health Examiners has found that the best walking pace is about 4 miles per hour. This is a brisk pace, amounting to about 15 minutes per mile. If you walk 3 miles at this pace, you should have 45 minutes in the target zone. Remember, most sedentary executives will not be able to keep up this pace without becoming exhausted. Begin your walking routine at a lower pace and work up to 4 miles per hour gradually.

Find a 1-mile stretch of street (you can use your car's odometer to measure it) and time yourself as you walk the distance at a brisk yet comfortable pace. You may be unable

[1] Charles T. Kuntzleman, *The Complete Book of Walking* (New York: Simon and Schuster, 1979), p. 21.
[2] Yehuda Shoenfeld, M.D., et al., "Walking: A Method for Rapid Improvement of Physical Fitness," *Journal of the American Medical Association*, May 23, 1980, pp. 2062–2063.

> # Running is such a jarring shock to the out-of-shape body that beginners should combine walking and running.

to walk that mile in 15 minutes, but that is perfectly all right. Just keep at it. If you do, you will find that after a few weeks you will be able to get to 4 miles per hour. You should also be checking your pulse to make sure your heartbeat is in the target zone.

As you begin to close in on a pace of 15 minutes per mile, your pulse should be reaching the target zone rapidly, and you should have little trouble keeping in the target zone for most of your walk. If your heartbeat is below your target zone level, you will need to build to a higher intensity. One way to do this is to increase your speed to a pace of five miles per hour (12 minutes per mile). Or as the Israeli study showed, you can carry a backpack or a briefcase. It usually takes from 4 to 6 weeks of walking for a previously inactive executive to reach the target zone rapidly.

Kuntzleman offers three more rules to follow to make sure you are walking at the proper intensity. First, you

IF YOU WANT TO KNOW MORE ABOUT WALKING

Contact the Walking Association, 4113 Lee Highway, Arlington, VA 22207 (phone: 703-527-5372). Two of the best overall books on walking are Charles T. Kuntzleman's *The Complete Book of Walking* (Simon and Schuster, 1979) and *The Magic of Walking* by Aaron Sussman and Ruth Goode (Simon and Schuster, 1967).

Dozens of books have been written in the last 5 years on the various aspects of running. Among the most comprehensive are James F. Fixx's *The Complete Book of Running* (Random House, 1977) and *Guidelines for Successful Jogging* [American Running and Fitness Association (formerly the National Jogging Association), 1977]. These and other books carry the same basic message for beginners: Beginners should start slowly and work their way up gradually, keeping alert to the body's danger signals, especially fatigue and muscle ache.

should be walking at a speed that will enable you to hold a conversation with someone beside you as you go. Second, you should have no pain while you walk. If you experience any sort of constant pain, see a doctor. Third, you should not be excessively tired after your walk. If you are, the walk was too strenuous, and you need to slow down. "All three points," Kuntzleman writes, "emphasize 'listening to your body.' This listening is something you'll have to learn. But you'll probably find it fun. You'll enjoy your body more. It will let you know when to slow down and when to speed up. You are the best judge of your exercise."[3]

Finally, Executive Health Examiners has found that walking helps eliminate executive stress for many of our patients. Also, walking sometimes is more effective in reducing stress than running. We think this is true because walkers travel at a more leisurely pace than runners. The walker therefore has the chance to enjoy the surroundings, drink in the ambience of a park, or feel the sunshine of a beautiful day.

Walking helps relieve stress in other ways. It is totally noncompetitive, for one thing, and it is a pastime that places no stress on any part of the body, including the mind. As one confirmed walker, the president of an accounting firm, told EHE doctors: "Now I know why Harry Truman took his 'daily constitutional.' My 45-minute walk from home to the office is the most relaxing thing I do all day. It sets my mind at ease and helps me get through the day. And after my walk home in the evening, I've left all the stresses of the office far behind me."

Running/Jogging

The first thing to remember about running or jogging (we use the words interchangeably because there is no clear distinction between the two; to see what the experts say, see Chapter 2) is that it can be hazardous to your health. Running is a strenuous form of exercise and demands a great deal from the body. If you are not in good shape, running can be a punishing activity, but it does not have to be. If you

[3] Charles T. Kuntzleman, *The Complete Book of Walking* (New York: Simon and Schuster, 1979), p. 93.

Calories Used Per Mile of Running

Weight	Number of minutes required to complete 1 mile		
	6	8	10
120	83	79	76
130	89	85	82
140	95	92	88
150	102	98	94
160	109	104	100
170	115	111	106
180	121	117	112
190	128	123	118
200	135	129	124
210	141	136	130
220	148	142	136

use common sense and take the proper precautions, you will find that running can be an exhilarating, stress-reducing, safe, and pleasurable experience.

Running presents a great potential danger to people with heart disease, which is why we strongly recommend that any executive over 35 have a complete physical examination including a stress test before setting out on a running program. Any executive under 35 who has been inactive for a long period of time should also have a physical examination before starting a jogging program.

With your doctor's consent, you can map out a running strategy. The first thing to do is to go out and spend a few dollars on a good sturdy pair of running shoes. We will give fuller details on the specifications for running shoes in Chapter 9. The most important thing to remember as you begin is to start *gradually*, especially if you have been living a sedentary life. Running is such a jarring shock to the out-of-shape body that Executive Health Examiners urges all beginners to combine walking and running at first and then to work gradually up to a total running regimen.

If you do not progress gradually, you run the risk of doing what one of our patients, a 41-year-old Connecticut

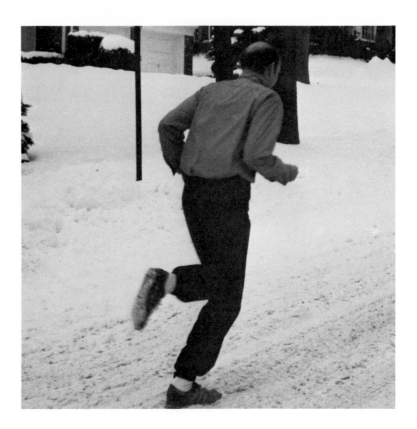

stockbroker, did several years ago. When this man began his program, he forced himself to run for 25 minutes five times a week. He refused to stop and walk when he became exhausted, because he felt he could not get enough benefit out of merely walking. Within a month, the bottoms of his feet were covered with blisters and his legs ached constantly. When he complained of his leg problems to EHE doctors, we asked about his running routine. When he told us what he had been doing, we suggested that he stop running until the blisters and other leg problems cleared up. He eventually began exercising again, but this time he started a routine of alternating running and walking. Two months later he was running again, and he had no leg problems.

Fixx writes:

It may take you several months to get to the point where you're running two, three or four miles at a time. Don't be in a hurry. Gradual improvement is safest. If you try to do too

Walking helps eliminate executive stress and can be more effective than running.

much too quickly, you're likely to hurt yourself. . . . If you find that your training increments are causing soreness or fatigue, slow your progress down.[4]

The American Running and Fitness Association concurs:

As much as we hate to hear it, those of us who are taking up this sport are no longer children. . . . Our "out-of-shape" condition quickly begins to show as we begin a new program. We become fatigued, get blisters, develop pains and pulls and strains, aches of all kinds. . . . In order to help you ambush their failure, consider the wisdom of the jogging motto of the Dolphin South End Runners of San Francisco, "Start slow and then taper off."[5]

Determining the best time of day to jog is entirely up to you. Whatever suits your schedule and sense of esthetics is best. The best place to jog is in a lightly wooded park with a running path, but you can jog just about anywhere: on city sidewalks, suburban streets, country roads, or running tracks. Running tracks provide the easiest way to keep a log of how many miles you run (just count the laps), but they also provide the highest potential of boring you to death as you continue to run in circles. Wherever you decide to run, try to make sure the surface is smooth. This will help avoid leg injuries.

A Beginner's Jogging Program

We recommend a 12-week beginner's jogging program of the American Running and Fitness Association. The sys-

---

[4] James Fixx, *The Complete Book of Running* (New York: Random House, 1977).

[5] *Guidelines for Successful Jogging* (The American Running and Fitness Association, formerly the National Jogging Association, 1977)

tem suggests distances for jogging and walking expressed not in miles but in minutes. These are guidelines; you may vary the distances to your taste, but try to stay within the general area. You should take an extra day of rest any time your body tells you to and feel free to substitute brisk walking for jogging at any point. Remember, after the first week or so, your primary objective is to get the heartbeat into the target zone for 20 to 30 minutes every time you run. Beginning in the second week, start checking your pulse fre-

WHEN YOU BEGIN TO JOG

First Week

Days 1, 3, and 5. Walk 15 minutes. Vary your pace. Try not to stop.

Days 2, 4, and 6. Walk 5 minutes, jog 1 minute, walk 5 minutes, jog 1 minute, walk 5 minutes. (Total time: 17 minutes)

Day 7. Rest.

Second Week

Days 1, 3, and 5. Walk 15 minutes, jog 1 minute.

Days 2, 4, and 6. Walk 5 minutes, jog 3 minutes, walk 5 minutes, jog 3 minutes, walk 5 minutes. (Total time: 21 minutes)

Day 7. rest.

Third Week

Days 1, 3, and 5. Walk 15 minutes, jog 1 minute.

Days 2, 4, and 6. Walk 6 minutes, jog 4 minutes, walk 6 minutes, jog 4 minutes, walk 6 minutes. (Total time: 26 minutes)

Day 7. Rest.

Fourth Week

Days 1, 3, and 5. Walk 15 minutes, jog 2 minutes.

Days 2, 4, and 6. Walk 3 minutes, jog 2 minutes. Repeat five more times. (Total time: 30 minutes)

Day 7. Rest.

Fifth Week

Days 1, 3, and 5. Walk 15 minutes, jog 2 minutes.
Days 2, 4, and 6. Walk 5 minutes, jog 5 minutes; repeat three times, ending with a 5-minute walk. (Total time: 35 minutes)
Day 7. Rest.

Sixth Week

Days 1, 3, and five. Walk 30 minutes.
Days 2, 4, and 6. Walk 4 minutes, jog 6 minutes; repeat twice more, ending with a 5-minute walk. (Total time: 35 minutes)
Day 7. Rest.

Seventh Week

Day 1. Walk for 30 minutes.
Days 2, 4, and 6. Walk 4 minutes, jog 6 minutes; repeat twice more, ending with a 5-minute walk. (Total time: 35 minutes)
Days 3 and 5. Walk 5 minutes, jog 10 minutes, walk 5 minutes.
Day 7. Rest.

Eighth Week

Day 1. Walk for 30 minutes.
Days 2, 4, and 6. Walk 2 minutes, jog 1 minute; repeat nine times, ending with a 5-minute walk. (Total time: 32 minutes)
Day 7. Rest.

Ninth Week

Days 1, 3, and 5. Walk 5 minutes, jog 1 minute, walk 1 minute. Repeat with 1 minute of each for 20 minutes. End with a 5-minute walk. (Total time: 30 minutes)
Day 7. Rest.

Tenth Week

Days 1, 3, and 5. Walk 5 minutes, jog 20 minutes, walk 5 minutes.

Days 2, 4, and 6. Walk 5 minutes, jog 10 minutes, walk 5 minutes.

Day 7. Rest.

Eleventh Week

Days 1, 3, and 5. Walk 5 minutes, jog 25 minutes, walk 5 minutes (always walk as needed).

Days 2, 4, and 6. Walk 5 minutes, jog 10 minutes, walk 5 minutes.

Day 7. Rest.

Twelfth Week

Days 1, 3, and 5. Walk 5 minutes, jog 30 minutes, walk 5 minutes.

Days 2, 4, and 6. Walk 5 minutes, jog 15 minutes, walk 5 minutes.

Day 7. Rest.

quently: before you start your run, 5 minutes or so after you have started running, and finally after you have finished. If you are below the target zone, increase the speed of your run or jog, but do not go over the target zone. If you feel yourself getting dizzy or if you have trouble catching your breath, slow down and then stop. Do not forget that the walking/jogging routine should be preceded by 10 to 15 minutes of warming up and followed by 10 to 15 minutes of cooling down.

It helps to keep a diary of your routine. Keep track of minutes, miles, and heartbeat and how you feel both physically and mentally. After you have completed the 12-week course, stay at the twelfth week's level for 4 more weeks. You will be ready to increase your distance when you feel no excessive fatigue or injury after your exercise. Move up about 10 percent at a time and stay at the new distance for at least 2 weeks before you go on.

For more details on this 12-week program, see the accompanying box, "When You Begin to Jog."

Cycling

Cycling is one of our recommended aerobic exercises that calls for the use of a major piece of equipment. For indoor cycling, you need a stationary bicycle; for outdoor riding, you need a simple three-speed bike. There are pluses and minuses involved in both indoor and outdoor cycling. By examining both routines, you can choose the one that suits you.

Outdoor Cycling

One prime advantage of cycling outdoors is that you can use your bike to commute to and from work. You can also take scenic rides and get aerobic exercise at the same time. But you cannot bicycle year-round in most climates, and bad weather at any time of the year can interrupt your cycling routine. You have to watch out for traffic if you ride in the streets. Pollution can be a problem in hot summer months, especially in large, congested cities. You must always keep in mind that bicycling can be dangerous; one spill, and you can injure yourself seriously. You also have to plan your route carefully to keep your heart in the target zone. Downhills and long flat stretches can cause you to ease up and fall below the target zone.

If after all those cautionary words you are still considering using an outdoor bicycling routine as your aerobic component, there is one more thing to keep in mind. We

A prime advantage of cycling is that you can use your bike to commute to and from work.

recommend that you have access to a bicycle path. If there is a bike path stretching from your house to near where you work, it's practically an invitation to pedal to and from work for aerobic exercise. You do not have to live within a few miles of the office to bicycle there and back. Remember the example of the publishing executive in Chapter 2 who lives 25 miles from the office. He puts his bike on the car and drives to within 5 miles of where he works. Then he parks the car, unhitches the bike, and pedals into work. He reverses the sequence in the evening.

Indoor Cycling

If you do not have a bike path readily available and want to cycle for aerobic exercise, consider purchasing a stationary bike. There are two big pluses with the indoor bike. First, you can cycle at any time of the year; weather is no inhibiting factor. Second, you can adjust the pedal resistance to a level at which your heartbeat will stay continuously in the target zone. The biggest drawback with the indoor cycle is that sitting and pedaling in the living room can be very boring. We saw in Chapter 3, though, how two executives surmounted that hurdle. One moved the television in front of her bike, and the other listened to tapes while pedaling.

Buying the Right Bicycle

If you decide to go with an outdoor cycling program, we recommend that you purchase a solid three-speed bicycle. If you prefer a five- or ten-speed bicycle, these have a range of low gears to enable you to flatten out hills without straining too much. Choose any major brand of bike from a reputable dealer. Before you leave the shop, make sure the salesperson adjusts the bicycle to fit your body. This is very important. The seat should be adjusted carefully for height so that when your leg is fully extended with your toe on the pedal, there will be a very slight bend in the knee. If the seat is too high or too low, you run the risk of injuring your knees. The seat also should be adjusted properly for distance from the handlebars. To do this, measure your arm's

IMPORTANCE OF PROPER SEAT ADJUSTMENT

(a) *Normal saddle height with foot at 6:30 (this number relates to the number on a clock), resulting in proper knee angle of 140° to 145°. (b) Saddle at position above normal, foot at 6:30, resulting in an increased knee angle of 160° to 165°. (c) Saddle at normal height with foot at 6:00 and knee angle of 145° to 150°, resulting in proper leg extension.*

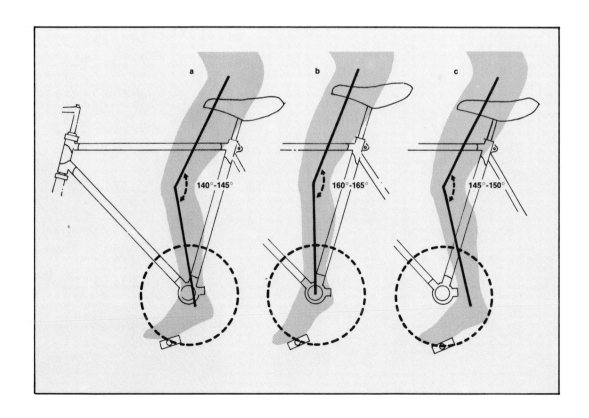

IMPORTANCE OF PROPER SEAT ADJUSTMENT (Cont.)

(a) Normal saddle height with foot at 12:00, resulting in proper knee angle of 65° to 70°. (b) Saddle at position below normal, resulting in a knee angle of less than 65°. (Source: J. Thomas Bohlmann, "Injuries in Competitive Cycling," The Physician and Sportsmedicine, May 1981.)

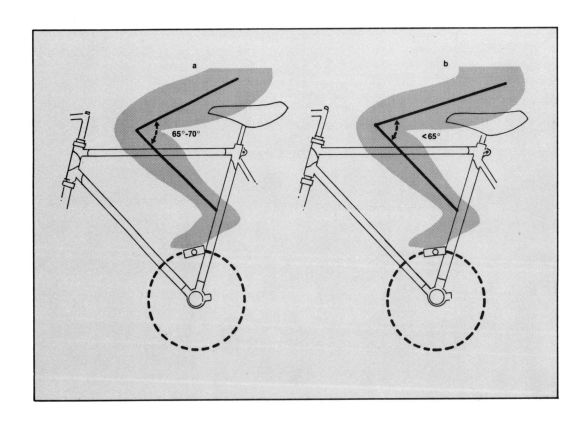

You can get the same aerobic benefit from the most simple bike that you can from the most complicated one.

length to the handlebars with your elbow resting in front of the seat. A properly adjusted seat enables you to ride in a relaxed and comfortable position.

The same basic rules apply when you are purchasing an indoor bike. There are dozens of types of indoor cycles on the market, from the simplest no-frills stationary bike to fancy ones that come with minicomputers to tell you what your pulse is each second, keep track of how much time you spent in the target zone, and automatically adjust the level of resistance of the pedals. The important thing to keep in mind is that you can get the same aerobic benefit from the most simple bike that you get from the most complicated.

The object is the same in cycling as it is in all aerobic exercise: to get your heartbeat in the target zone for 20 to 30 minutes at least three times a week. It's up to you to decide what type of stationary bike to buy. The only mandatory criteria are that the seat be adjustable so that the fit is perfect for your body, that the bike be sturdy and not wobble or make excessive noise, and that it be equipped with an easily adjustable device to vary pedal resistance. It also helps to have a speedometer.

The routine for both indoor and outdoor bicycling is the same as in all other aerobic exercises. Before you start, spend about 5 minutes warming up with stretches and calisthenics. Pay particular attention to the leg muscles; make sure they are well stretched out before you get on the bike. Unlike running, cycling causes no harsh jolting to the legs. You do need strong leg muscles to cycle steadily for long distances, but you can build up those muscles through a combination of isometric and isotonic exercises and your aerobic cycling regimen.

Once you get on the bike, take it easy for the first 5 minutes or so. This is considered a warmup time. When you have loosened up, start pedaling harder for 5 minutes and then check your pulse. If you are not up to the target zone, try pedaling a bit faster. After 20 minutes in the target zone, begin gearing down and pedal lightly for 5 to 10 minutes to cool off. When you get off the bike, stretch out again for a final cooling-off minute.

If you have been sedentary for a long time, it is wise to proceed extremely cautiously for the first few weeks of cycling. You can even forget about the target zone for the first 2 weeks. Just concentrate on pedaling up to a speed that feels comfortable without overexerting yourself. After you are used to the feel of the bike, begin checking your pulse and adjusting your speed and intensity to get in the target zone for 20 to 30 minutes per session.

In *The Complete Book of Bicycling*, Eugene A. Sloan gives the outline of a recommended routine on an outdoor bike for the sedentary executive:

> Keep your bicycle in the lowest, or next to lowest gear and ride slowly, without strain, three or four miles a day for two or three weeks. Build up your cycling stamina gradually by increasing your daily rides by two or three miles each week. If you are in good health . . . you will probably find that ten miles or so a day will keep you fit and trim.

Swimming

Swimming is the only aerobic activity recommended by Executive Health Examiners that requires facilities not available in most homes. If you decide to choose swimming as your aerobic exercise, you are going to have to make ar-

Swimming, unlike other regimens, exercises all the body's muscle groups, including the arms, trunk, and legs.

rangements to travel to and from a swimming pool that has time set aside for lap swimming. This does not necessarily have to take up large amounts of your time. Many executives find that swimming is a perfect lunch-hour activity. The research director of a hospital in New York City, for example, lives thirty blocks from his YMCA swimming pool, but the pool is only two blocks from his office. He takes a 5-minute walk to the Y at noontime three days a week, depending on his schedule, and thereby receives an aerobic workout without interrupting his everyday routine.

There are other ways to get in your swimming without taking too much time from your daily activities. You can stop off at the pool on the way to work or on the way home. Either way, you will take about 90 minutes out of your day. This is an hour and a half that is especially well spent, because of the extra benefits of swimming. Swimming, of course, fulfills the aerobic component of your exercise regimen. But swimming, unlike walking, running, or cycling, also exercises all the body's muscle groups, including the arms, trunk, and legs. Another attribute of swimming is that it is the only one of the recommended aerobic programs that is not weight-bearing. In walking, cycling, and especially running, the legs bear the brunt of the exercise. However, in swimming the water holds you up, and very little strain is put on the ankles and knees. This is why we especially recommend swimming for those with ankle or knee injuries and for older persons. It is not uncommon to see men and women in their sixties and seventies and older slowly but steadily swimming laps at many pools.

There is one final aspect of swimming that should help you decide whether it is the right aerobic exercise for you. If you are not comfortable in the water, if you do not like water sports, or if you can swim but are not very good at it (if you flail around, expending a lot of energy but getting nowhere fast), we suggest that you consider another aerobic activity. This is not to say that only polished swimmers should take up swimming as an aerobic exercise, but it certainly bodes well for your future happiness in the water if you already have a modicum of swimming ability.

If you have decided that swimming is right for you, here are some hints on how to get started. First, find a 20- or 25-

Rope skipping is not for everyone. In fact, it is so strenuous that some doctors do not recommend it for the average sedentary person.

yard pool that is close to your home or office. Then examine your daily schedule and find the best time to fit in a swimming routine. You will need only one piece of equipment, a bathing suit. If you have sensitive eyes, you may want to purchase a pair of swimmer's goggles, which, by the way, can be ordered with prescription lenses.

A Swimming Regimen

The routine for your swimming exercise has the same basic outline as the routine for other aerobic programs. You need a warmup, 20 to 30 minutes of aerobic activity, and then a cooling-down period. As with cycling, most of your warmup and cooling-down time can come during the beginning and end of aerobic activity.

Begin with a few minutes of stretching exercises before you get in the pool. Then swim a lap and check your pulse. Most pools have a large swim clock on hand so that you will not need to wear your watch in the pool. After another warmup lap or two, check your pulse again. Take a few more laps and recheck your pulse. Here's the advice of Dr. Lenore Zohman about pulse taking and the beginning swimming regimen: "Your carotid pulse rate and your feeling of tiredness can tell you whether you are doing too little or too much and, over the next few days and weeks, whether you are making progress. If you can cover more laps at the same pulse rate, you are getting there."[6]

We recommend that beginners use just one stroke. Try the overhand crawl, the least demanding stroke. As in all

[6] Lenore Zohman, et al., *The Cardiologists' Guide to Fitness and Health through Exercise* (New York: Simon and Schuster, 1979).

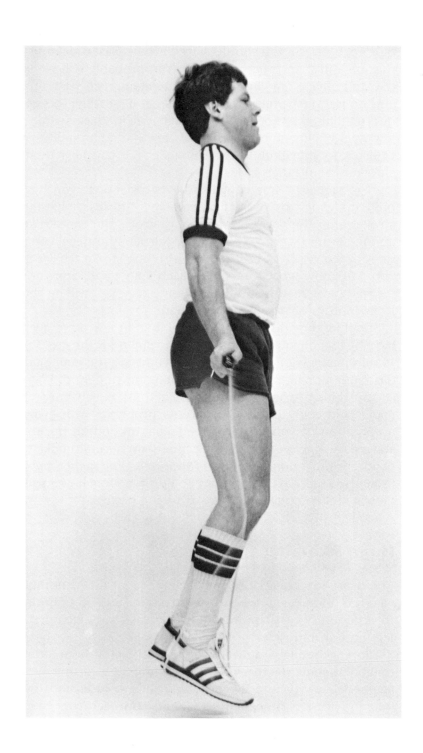

types of exercise, you should start with the least demanding routine and then progress slowly. You probably will be exhausted after a few laps at first. Therefore, take your time and do not push yourself. If you keep at it steadily, you will find that your cardiovascular capacity will increase within a few weeks. Remember to progress slowly and gradually and to listen to your body for warning signs. If you hear them, slow down and then stop.

You can experiment with other strokes after you have built up your cardiovascular capacity. The least vigorous strokes after the crawl are the breaststroke, the backstroke, and the butterfly. Once you attain proficiency and feel confident in the pool, it's best to stay with one stroke. That way you will know what it takes to reach your target zone and will not have to stop and check your pulse. You will be able to feel intuitively when you are there.

Cooling down is easier in a pool than in any other aerobic activity. All you have to do is slow down for the last 5 to 10 minutes of your program. Before you leave the pool, paddle about for a bit to finish your cooling-down period. There is no problem with getting overheated, because the water cools your body and also prevents problems with sweat evaporation. If you want more details on setting up and staying in a swimming routine, there are several books to choose from. Among the best is *Swimming For Total Fitness* (1980) by Jane Katz and Nancy P. Burning, which provides details of a complete aerobic swimming program.

Rope Skipping

The main advantage of rope skipping is that it is extremely vigorous and gets your heart to the target zone very rapidly. In addition, rope skipping helps increase strength in the legs and arm muscles.

Rope skipping is not for everyone. In fact, it is so strenuous that some doctors do not recommend it for the average sedentary person. Recent studies have indicated that people with low fitness levels should approach rope skipping with extreme caution, since it taxes the body so enormously in a brief period of time.

It was once thought that 10 minutes of rope skipping provided the same cardiovascular benefits as 30 minutes of running, but a recent study found that the claim is "exaggerated and unfounded" and that "the energy requirement imposed by skipping rope is not reasonable for the average sedentary person."[7]

Because rope skipping is so easy to do, takes only one piece of equipment, and can be done just about anywhere, we recommend it. But there is an important caveat: Undertake rope skipping only after a physical examination by a doctor that includes a stress test, and make sure you specifically ask the doctor for permission to set out on a rope-skipping exercise program.

If you have your doctor's permission, remember that the same rules of warmup, 20 to 30 minutes in the target zone, and a period of cooling down apply in rope skipping. When you start, begin extremely gradually and be cautious at all times for signs of exhaustion. Do not overstrain. At the first sign of fatigue, stop.

[7] Bud Getchell, Ph.D., and Pat Clearly, M.A., "The Caloric Costs of Rope Skipping and Running," *The Physician and Sportsmedicine*, February 1980, p. 60.

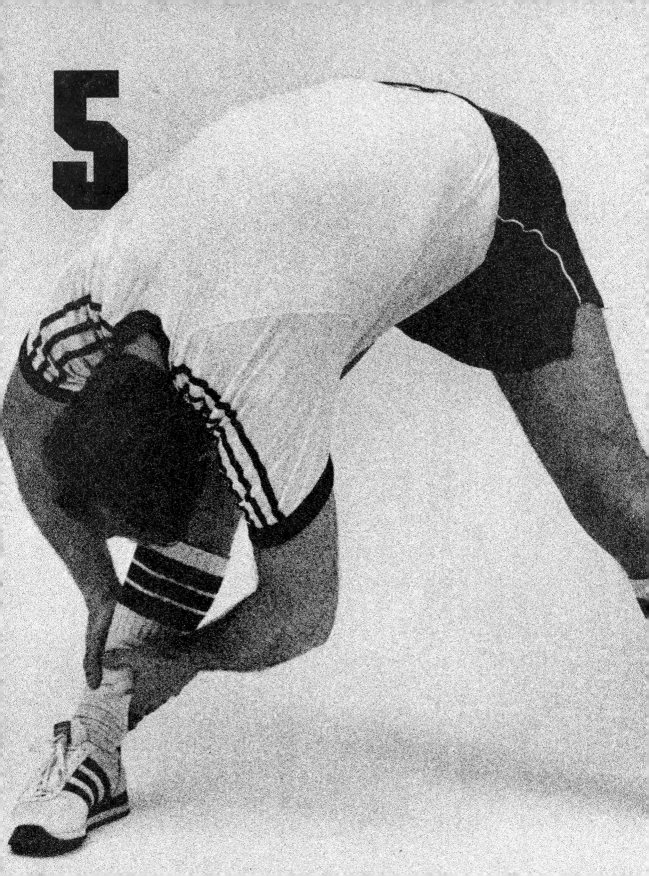

STRENGTH BUILDING AND STRETCHING: COMPLEMENTS TO AEROBICS

There are two other components that round out the EHE total fitness program: strength-building and stretching exercises. As we pointed out in Chapters 3 and 4, aerobic exercises should be the key element of your exercise regimen, but for total fitness you must also build up strength and at the same time keep your muscles stretched out and flexible.

You will have to work on the muscles three to five times a week, spending 10 to 15 minutes per session on the stretching exercises and another 10 to 15 minutes on the strength-building routines. You have the option of doing these exercises separately or integrating them into your aerobic sessions during the warmup and cooling-down periods. These exercises complement each other, and they also complement the aerobic exercises, since strong and flexible muscles enable you to walk, run, cycle, swim, or skip rope without putting undue strain on your musculoskeletal system. Well stretched out muscles provide an extra bonus by helping to reduce the possibility of injury and easing physical tension. In so doing, they can help you soothe the stress of mental tension as well.

Strength-Building Exercises

Just as aerobic exercises in effect build up the heart muscles, strength-building exercises build up another set of muscles, the skeletal muscles. The strength-building exercises have almost no direct effect on the cardiovascular system, but they are important in an overall fitness regimen for two reasons. First, they help you perform aerobic routines more easily. Second, strong muscles help in everyday activities such as moving, lifting, and holding weight. By building strength in the 400-odd skeletal muscles you will be able to perform any number of tasks—from lifting a suitcase off a baggage rack to pushing your lawn mower—without strain or discomfort. Having strong muscles also gives you a subtle but palpable feeling of confidence in your physical capabilities.

The strength-building exercises are in some ways similar to the aerobic exercises; both involve pushing muscles to perform beyond their normal capacity. Then, between exercise sessions, the resting muscles increase in strength. However, there is also a fundamental difference between aerobic and strength-building exercises.

In aerobics you push the cardiovascular system to work at a level of 70 to 85 percent of maximal heart capacity (the

Having strong muscles gives you a subtle but palpable feeling of confidence in your physical capabilities.

target zone), but strength-building exercises require you to push your muscles to their maximum. In other words, in strength building you overload the muscles to force them to work as hard as they can. In both types of exercises the muscles reset themselves between sessions so that they can perform more demanding tasks.

The Risk of Injury

As you might expect, pushing muscles to their limit involves some risk of injury, especially for sedentary individuals. Thus, common sense dictates that when you begin a strength-building program, you should start gradually, progress slowly, and be alert for signs of danger.

The main danger for a sedentary executive embarking on a program of weight lifting, situps, pushups, chinups, or other strength-building activities involves blood pressure. These exercises increase blood pressure, making the heart work harder as its need for oxygen increases. When this happens, the blood flow to the heart and brain can be reduced, and the cardiovascular system can be endangered. Therefore, if you think you have any of the risk factors associated with coronary disease (obesity, high blood pressure, high cholesterol, or cigarette smoking), or if you have been sedentary for a long time, it is wise to consult a doctor before beginning a program of strength-building exercises. This also holds true for anyone with known heart disease.

After securing your physician's permission, it still is best to proceed extremely cautiously. One important thing to keep in mind is not to hold your breath when you lift, push, and strain. You should breathe freely and deeply, concentrating on exhaling forcefully when you are putting out the most effort, like the karate experts who let out loud screams as they smash bricks with their hands.

Isometrics, Isotonics, and Calisthenics

Isometrics refers to a type of strength-building exercise that gained some popularity in the 1950s and 1960s. In isometric exercises you build up muscles by exerting pressure against an immovable object. This high-intensity exercise builds strength and muscle tone when the muscle contracts as you exert considerable force for only 6 to 10 seconds. These exercises include pushing against a wall, doorjamb, chair, or desk. After several weeks of steady practice, you can make substantial improvement in muscle strength and tone.

But isometric exercises have significant drawbacks, and Executive Health Examiners recommends them only to those very few persons who cannot spare 10 to 15 minutes three times a week to do other strength-building exercises. One problem with isometric exercises is that each exercise benefits only one muscle. This makes it nearly impossible to devise a balanced isometric strength-building program. You would need dozens of individual isometric exercises to build strength in all the leg, arm, back, and shoulder muscles. Moreover, isometric exercises require such concentrated intensity that we do not recommend them for people with cardiovascular risk factors. Executive Health Examiners agrees with the American College of Sports Medicine, which discourages isometrics both for sedentary persons and for those with cardiac disease risk factors.

The bottom line on isometric exercises is that if you feel you must do them, check with your doctor, especially if you are leading a sedentary life. Then proceed slowly and cautiously, remembering to breathe deeply while you exercise. You should also devise a routine in which many different muscles from all the major muscle groups are involved.

Since isometric exercises can be performed almost anywhere and at any time, you can do them on the train or bus as you commute to and from the office. You can even do

You should devise a routine which involves many different muscles from all the major muscle groups.

With any exercise routine, be alert to signs from your body.

them in your office whenever you need a short break during the day.

There is no set order for isometric exercises, and you do not have to do an entire routine in one session. You can therefore spice up different parts of the day by taking 2- or 3-minute isometric breaks.

Isometric exercises require concentrated effort, but you should not hold any one contraction longer than 8 seconds; 6 seconds is all that is necessary. When you first begin isometric exercises, it's best to take it easy and hold off giving your maximum effort for about 3 or 4 weeks. During that initial time, expend only about half your maximum force. During the first 3 or 4 seconds of each exercise, build up to your maximal effort—or half maximum when you are just starting out—and for the final 3 or 4 seconds, maintain that intensity. You should gradually increase your effort in the fourth and fifth weeks so that by the sixth week you can give maximum effort for the full 6 to 8 seconds you do each isometric exercise.

As with any exercise routine, be alert to signs from your body. If you experience pain, your muscles are telling you they cannot handle the intensity. Cut back on your effort immediately. If the pain persists, stop doing the particular exercise for a few weeks. When you go back, take it easy at first and then stop at the first sign of pain.

Here are eight isometric exercise routines that strengthen the neck, upper body, arms, chest, abdomen, lower back, buttocks, thighs, and legs. Remember to relax and breathe deeply between exercises and not to hold the contractions longer than 8 seconds. Remember, at the first sign of pain, immediately stop and forget about doing that exercise for a while.

The Neck

Isometric exercises for the neck are done in a sitting or standing position with the fingers interlaced on the forehead. The idea is to push your head forward while at the same time pushing back equally hard with the hands. The counterexercise is done with the fingers interlaced behind the head. You push the head back and the hands forward. To exercise the sides of the neck, place the palm of the left hand on the left side of the head and push with the hand while resisting with the head and the neck. Do the same with the right hand on the right side of the head.

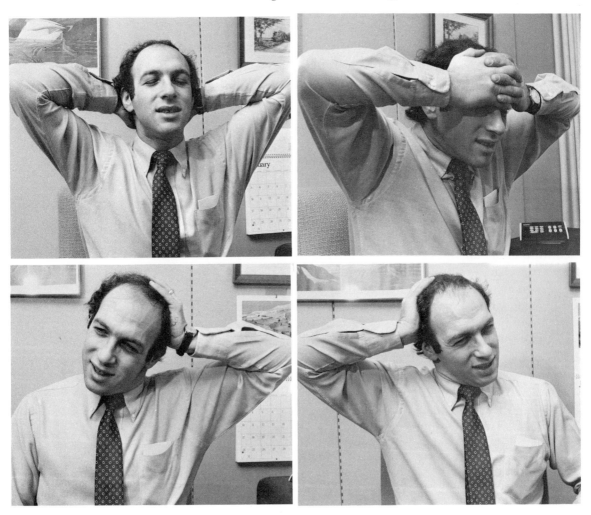

The Upper Body

The first isometric exercise for the upper body is done in a standing position with your back to the wall. Put your hands at your sides, palms against the wall, and press your hands backward against the wall. Keep your arms straight. Then face the wall with your hands at your sides, palms against the wall, and press forward, keeping your arms straight. Finally, stand in a doorway or with your side against a wall and your right palm facing your right leg. Press your right hand outward against the wall or doorframe, keeping the arm straight. Repeat with the left arm.

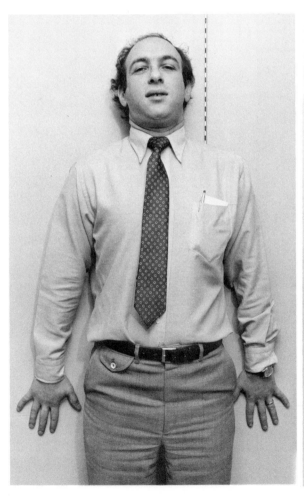 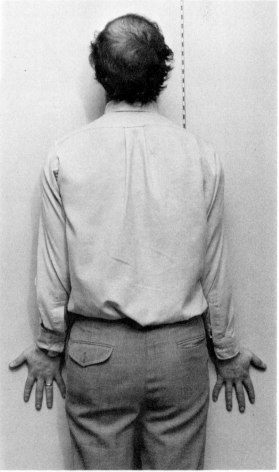

The Arms

For the arms, stand with your feet about 12 inches apart. First flex your right elbow close to your body with the palm up. Then put your left hand on top of your right hand in front of you and forcibly try to curl your right arm up while pushing down with the left hand. Then repeat with the left arm and the right hand.

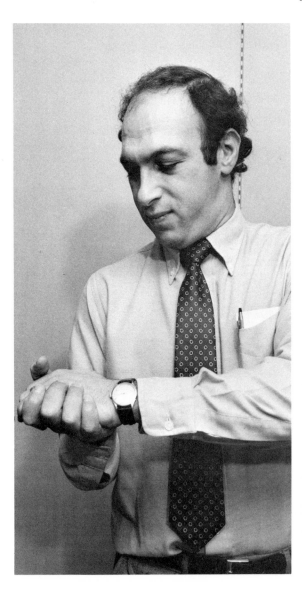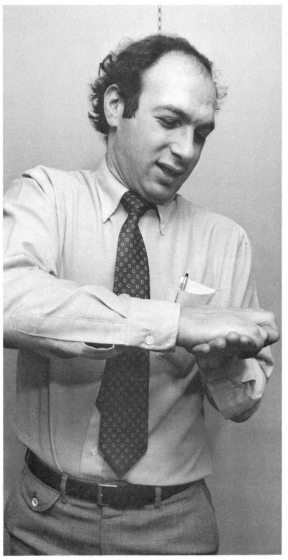

The Chest

To strengthen the arms and chest at the same time, stand with your feet a shoulder length apart and your knees slightly bent. Clasp your hands with the palms together close to your chest; then press the hands together. Hold for 6 to 8 seconds. Now grip your fingers together with your arms in the same position and pull hard.

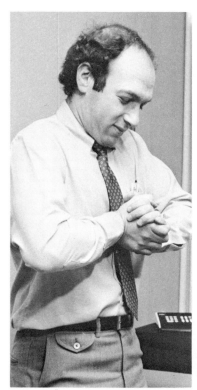
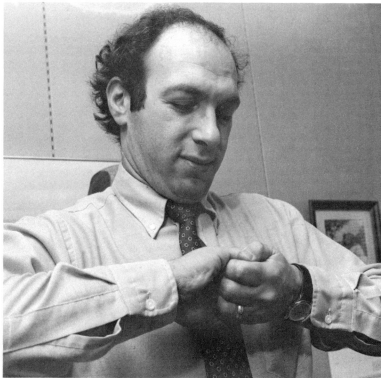

The Abdomen

For the abdominal muscles, stand with your knees slightly bent and your hands resting on the tops of your knees. Forcibly contract your abdominal muscles for the required 6 to 8 seconds.

The Lower Back, Buttocks, and Thighs

To strengthen the lower back, buttocks, and the backs of the thighs, lie face down on the floor with your arms at your sides, palms down. Maneuver your legs under a table, chair, desk, or other heavy object. With the hips flat on the floor raise one leg, keeping the knee straight. Make sure the heel is pushing hard against the table or chair. Hold for 6 to 8 seconds, and then repeat with the opposite leg.

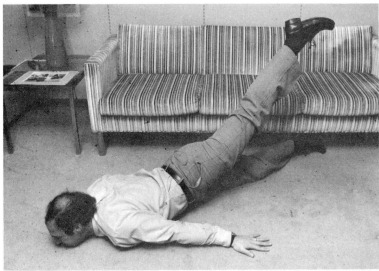

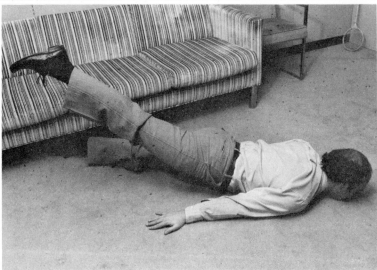

The Legs

The best isometric exercises for the leg muscles are done sitting in a chair. Cross the left ankle over the right with your feet on the floor and your legs bent at a 90 degree angle. Try with all your might to straighten your right leg while resisting the push with your left. Repeat with the opposite legs.

The inner thigh muscles can be strengthened isometrically by sitting in a chair and extending your legs with each ankle pressed against the outside of another chair's legs. Make sure the second chair is sturdy. Keep the legs straight and pull one toward the other. To exercise the outer thighs, put your ankles inside the chair legs and exert pressure outward.

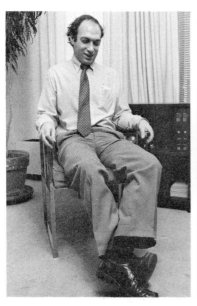 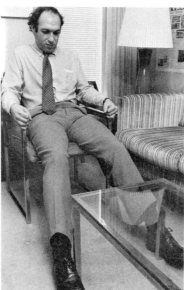 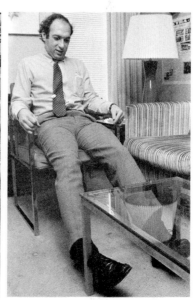

The Isotonic Alternative

A much better all-around program for strengthening muscles is provided by isotonic exercises. Isotonic exercises include weight lifting as well as calisthenics such as pushups and situps. It's quite easy to incorporate a few isotonic exercises into your regular aerobic routine during the 10- to 15-minute warmup and cooling-down periods.

A Beginner's Calisthenics Routine

Here is a calisthenics routine to use for either warming up or cooling down in conjunction with aerobic exercise. If you use these calisthenics for cooling down, give yourself a few minutes of rest after completing your run, walk, swim, or cycling. The last part of your aerobic routine should be done in slow motion; that is, if you have just finished running, walk slowly but steadily for about 5 minutes. Spend the last few minutes of cycling or swimming taking it very easy and then gradually slow to a halt. Then take some deep breaths and stretch your arms and legs gradually. Limber up a bit before beginning, swinging your arms from side to side, shaking out your legs and arms, and rolling your head and neck in circles.

Now you are ready to do calisthenics. We recommend starting with side stretches to tone your midsection. Stand with your feet a shoulder length apart and your hands clasped behind your head. Bend to the left as far as possible, hold that position for a second, and then return to the starting point. Bend to the right and repeat left and right fifteen to twenty times.

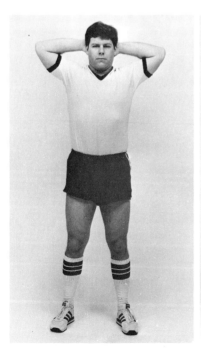 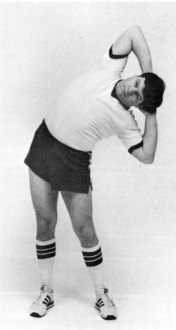 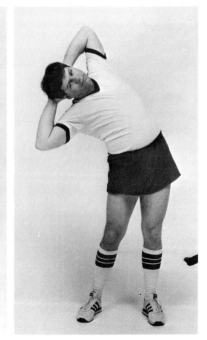

Situps

The next exercises are situps. There are many ways to do situps, which strengthen the abdominal and back muscles. You can keep your knees bent or extend them out straight. You can sit on a slant board or raise your legs up on a chair. You can touch your right elbow to your left knee and then your left elbow to your right knee. You can clasp your hands behind your head, keep them at your sides, or stretch them over your head. You can come halfway up, sit up just enough to see your toes, or come all the way up and touch the toes. Choose the routine that is right for you, one you can do without undue strain but one that also requires some effort. It is recommended that individuals with low back disorders perform situps with knees bent, since this technique places less strain on the back.

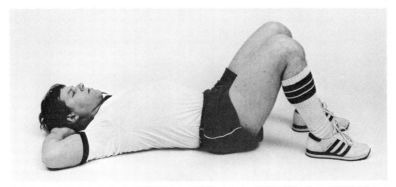

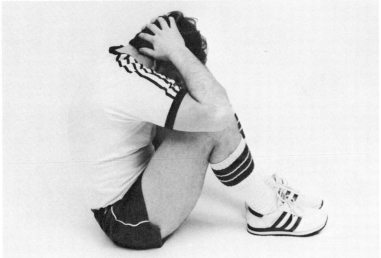

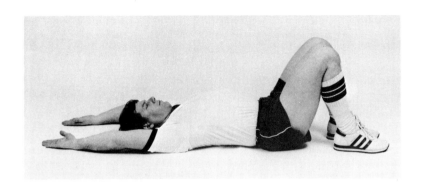

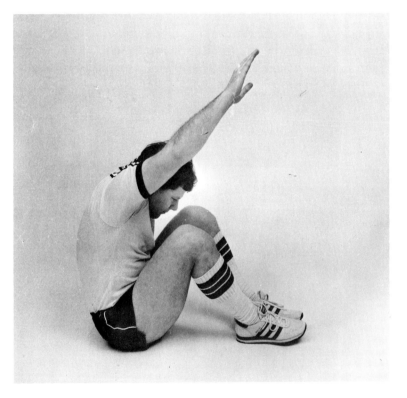

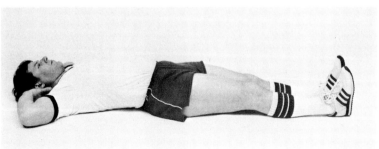

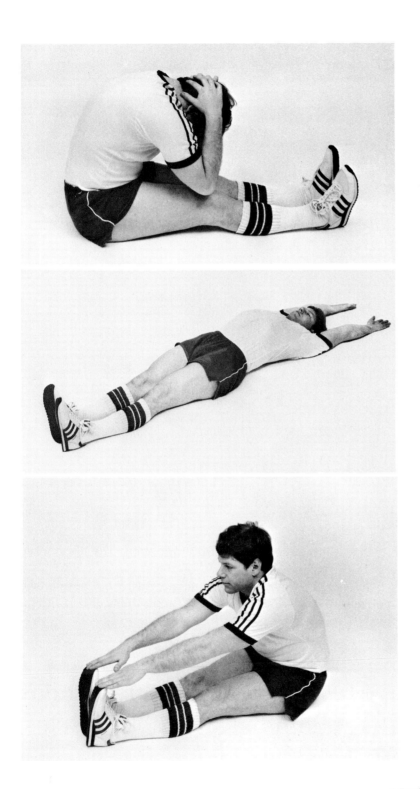

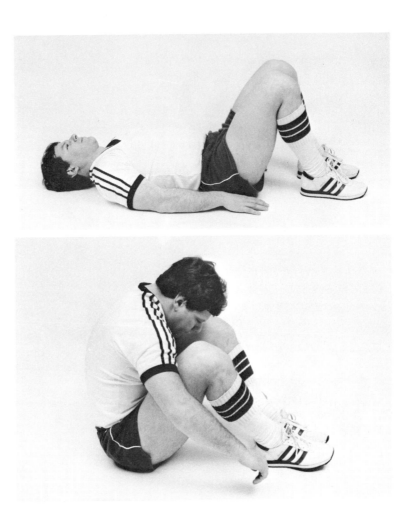

Each different type of situp strengthens the abdominal and back muscles.

If you are really out of shape, start with ten situps and then add one or two a week until you hit thirty. If you can do thirty situps easily, try for fifty.

Each type of situp strengthens the abdominal and back muscles.

Pushups

After your situps, take a minute to stretch out. Take some deep breaths. Now you are ready for the pushup routine, an excellent strength builder for the shoulders, chest, and back of the arms. Pushups are hard work. You may have trouble doing even one or two, but keep at it. If you practice regularly, you will see dramatic improvement in weeks. Try for a maximum of thirty pushups at one time. When you reach thirty—and this may take 6 months or longer—stay with it.

A good pushup goes like this: Keep the body straight; do not sag and do not arch your back. Keep the legs together. Put your palms on the floor and keep them a couple of inches outside your shoulders. Your weight should be distributed evenly between your hands and toes. Keeping your body in a straight line, push up until the elbows are straight. Then let yourself down to the point where your nose or forehead brushes the floor. Do not let your stomach or chest hit the floor. Then push up again.

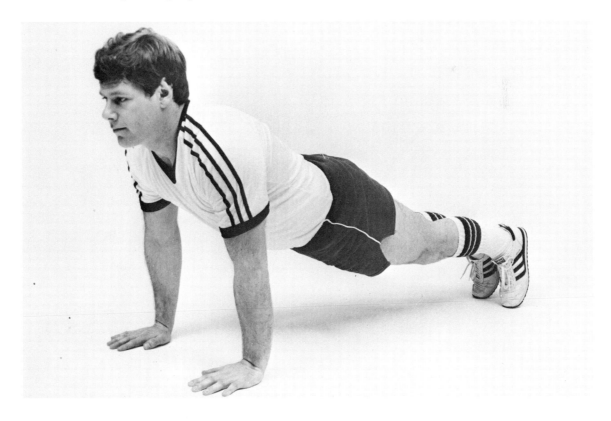

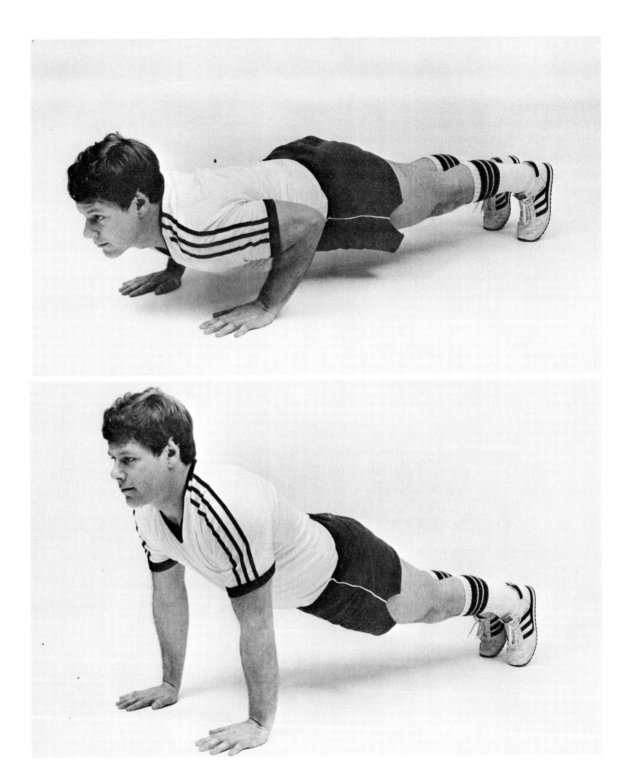

If you cannot do one regular pushup, try modified pushups, in which you keep the knees on the floor and push with your hands. If you keep at this for a few weeks, you will soon develop the strength to do regular pushups.

If thirty regular pushups a day are easy for you, there are ways to make them a bit more challenging. Try fingertip, or "Marine," pushups, in which you clap your hands between each push. We have found that for most executives, thirty pushups three times a week is sufficient to get good muscle strength and tone in the upper body.

Pullups

The final calisthenic is the pullup. For this you need a sturdy steel pullup bar, which can be mounted in almost any doorway, at home or in the office. There are various pullup (sometimes called chinup) methods, all of which build strong arm and shoulder muscles as you lift all your weight with the upper body.

Some executives cannot do even one pullup the first time. The secret is to keep plugging and not give up. It is simply a matter of time before the muscles gain enough strength to do the job of pulling your chin up to the bar. Once you are able to do one pullup, you will feel a sense of accomplishment, and soon you will be doing two or three. Aim for sets of six pullups. When that gets easy, go for sets of ten. Do no more than three sets per warmup or cooling-down period.

If you are interested in doing an extra abdominal muscle-building routine at the same time you do pullups, try leg lifts on the pullup bar. Pull yourself up on the bar and hang there for a moment with your chin over the bar. Then try to bring both legs up parallel with the floor without bending your knees. Hold the legs out there for a second and then let them down slowly. Do not swing the legs for momentum; make your stomach and back muscles do the work. Try for sets of six, and if you find that easy, do sets of ten.

These calisthenics provide a well-rounded strength-building routine that takes only about 15 minutes per session. If you do this routine three times a week, you will see improvements in overall body strength in a matter of months.

Weight Lifting and Calisthenics

The main difference between weight training and calisthenics is that weight lifting builds up muscular strength in a few specific muscles, while calisthenics exercises provide strength to a range of muscles. Executive Health Examiners does not recommend weight lifting for most executives. However, if you need to strengthen certain muscles that have atrophied from longtime neglect, if you need to build up leg or arm muscles to be more proficient in your aerobic routine, or if you merely want to build overall body strength, a weight-training program could be the answer.

Such a program will take up a lot of your time. You will need to spend a minimum of 30 minutes on each weight-training session. An ideal session should last about 90 minutes and should consist of ten to twenty different exercises designed to build up the muscles in all parts of the body. You should work out every other day. You can combine weight training and aerobic exercises in one session, but this would lengthen your total exercise period by at least a half hour—probably by as much as an hour—and most executives cannot spare that amount of time on a regular basis.

The Benefits of Calisthenics

We believe the best way to include strength-building exercises in your fitness routine is to incorporate calisthenics into your warmup and cooling-down periods before and after an aerobic walking, running, swimming, cycling, or rope-skipping session. Calisthenics fits in well with aerobics because calisthenics involves low-level muscular strength-building exercises that, unlike isometric exercises, put very little stress on the circulatory system. Yet calisthenics works efficiently to strengthen the muscles.

Calisthenic exercises therefore present few problems for sedentary executives or those with cardiac disease risk factors, although commonsense precautions should be taken while performing calisthenics, just as with any other type of exercise.

Calisthenic exercises such as pushups, situps, jumping jacks, and pullups work well as warmups for running, walking, and cycling because they get the heart moving while at the same time exercising the upper-body muscles. An ideal exercise program combines calisthenics, some isotonics, and a series of stretching exercises wrapped around your aerobic routine.

For a program combining all three forms of exercises, see the accompanying box, "Total Fitness on an Exercise Trail."

TOTAL FITNESS ON AN EXERCISE TRAIL

There is a form of activity that combines in one session all the needed components of a total fitness regimen: stretching, strength building, and aerobics. It is the exercise trail, also known by the trade name Parcourse. The exercise trail was invented in Switzerland and was brought to this country in 1973. Since then, many trails have been installed in parks throughout the country, from Rock Creek Park in Washington, D.C., to the San Francisco Bay course in the shadow of the Golden Gate Bridge.

A typical exercise trail has from fifteen to twenty points. Each point contains a printed set of instructions which tells you what stretching or strength-building exercise to do and suggests routines for beginning, intermediate, and advanced participants. The idea is to walk, jog, or cycle the 100 to 250 yards between stations. The printed instructions range from simple signs telling you how to stretch the hamstring muscles to slant boards for situps and bars of different heights for chinups.

If you are lucky enough to live or work near an exercise course, try it out. It's doubtful you will be able to use it for your regular exercise routine—primarily because you cannot run through the course in inclement weather—but a weekly, biweekly, or even monthly run through a fitness course will provide a welcome break from your regular exercise program. Besides, it's fun.

Stretching helps impart a feeling of calmness to the body and the mind.

Stretching for Flexibility

Stretching exercises are an integral part of the EHE fitness routine. Stretching provides a kind of preventive maintenance for the muscles. It helps loosen tight muscles that can cause injuries such as cramps, strains, and pulls. Stretching exercises also help relieve tension in the muscles. In so doing, they also relieve other kinds of bodily tension, including mental stress. Stretching helps impart a feeling of calmness to the body and the mind.

Stretching exercises can make up the bulk of your warmup routine. For those who run, walk, or cycle, the leg muscles—especially the thighs, calves, and Achilles tendons—must be loose and stretched out. The important thing to remember when stretching for flexibility is to perform the exercises very slowly and progress gradually. Stretch the muscles slowly, relax for a few seconds, and then stretch slowly again until you feel the tenseness ease.

The Art of Yoga

Some of the most beneficial stretching exercises were developed as part of the ancient Indian system of exercise called yoga, but many executives seem to have a mental block against yoga. When they hear the word, it brings visions of exoticism, although nothing could be further from the truth. As executives who have taken our advice and joined yoga classes have found, yoga is a demanding form of exercise that requires coordination, flexibility, and strength.

One EHE client, a 43-year-old Connecticut bank vice

president, took his first yoga class 4 years ago at the suggestion of a friend. A yoga center near his office offered open classes at noontime five days a week, and he decided to try a class one Wednesday afternoon. The first class was torture; he could not seem to bring his stiff limbs into any of the pretzel-like postures. But this man felt very relaxed after that first session and decided to try it again the next week. He has continued going to noontime sessions nearly every week since then, and he also does yoga stretches every morning at home. On the three mornings a week when he runs, he does an abbreviated yoga routine, including the twelve-part salute to the sun, which is discussed later in this chapter, a perfect warmup exercise for aerobics because it stimulates nearly every muscle in the body. On days when he does not run, he does a 45-minute routine that mixes yoga with some calisthenics.

To find out about yoga, enroll in a special beginner's class or at a health club, yoga school, or adult-education class. Or, as the Connecticut banker did, you can join an open class, one that is open to beginners, intermediate, and advanced yoga practitioners. After you have learned the basics, you can do an entire routine (or a few postures of your choice) at any time and place. Yoga requires no equipment or facilities not found in the home. A well-padded rug and some loose exercise clothing (or a leotard) are all you need.

Yoga can help any sedentary executive not only to stretch his or her muscles but also to relax. As your yoga instructor will no doubt tell you, relaxation is as important as exercising during a yoga routine. You make a conscious effort between postures to relax your mind and body. Taking the time to do yoga during the middle of a hectic day is a good antidote to the tensions and pressures inherent in the executive lifestyle, and a yoga class at noon can be a refreshing change from a three-martini lunch.

A Beginner's Yoga Program

Here is a yoga program you can do on your own in the morning before you leave for the office, in the evening after the hectic events of the day, or even during your lunch break.

All you need is a room with a well-padded rug, a sheet, a blanket or mat, and some loose clothing. This yoga routine lasts about 40 minutes, but if you are in a hurry, you can cut it to a half hour. Even if you are trying to cut the routine to 30 minutes, take things slowly while doing the exercises. You can gain time by cutting down on the rest periods between exercises.

Remember, during the entire session breathe deeply from the diaphragm, the area where your chest and abdominal cavity meet. Also, be sure to breathe through your nose with your mouth closed. Deep breathing is an important part of the yoga routine. It helps relax the body and enables you to stretch the muscles without undue discomfort. By concentrating on your breath before, during, and after the yoga exercises, you help yourself relax and enable the muscles to stretch out and become more flexible.

To start the routine, sit with your eyes closed (this will help you concentrate on the task at hand and shut out all extraneous thoughts) in a comfortable cross-legged position. Relax while at the same time sitting up straight. Take

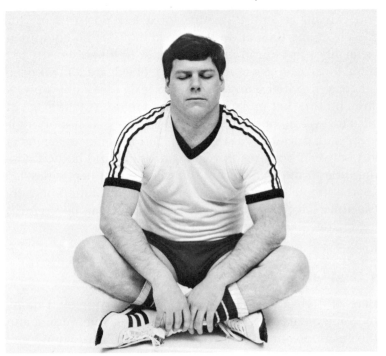

several deep breaths from the diaphragm, counting slowly to 4 as you inhale, holding the breath for four counts, and exhaling for another 4 seconds. With diaphragmatic breathing, as you inhale, your stomach expands like a balloon; as you exhale, your stomach deflates.

Take six to eight of these deep breaths and concentrate on the ebbing and flowing of air through your body. Try to block out all other thoughts. Let your breathing return to normal; then relax with your eyes closed for a minute or two. This simple relaxing meditative breathing will get your mind and body ready to begin the yoga exercises, which are called postures or poses.

Neck Rolls The first few yoga exercises are warmups. Begin with neck rolls. With your eyes closed for concentration, drop your chin slowly to your chest and then bring it back to center. Hold that for a second and then let your head fall back as far as you can without overstraining. Repeat this back and forth motion four more times, coordinating the neck movements with the breath.

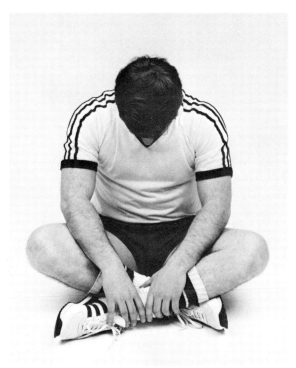
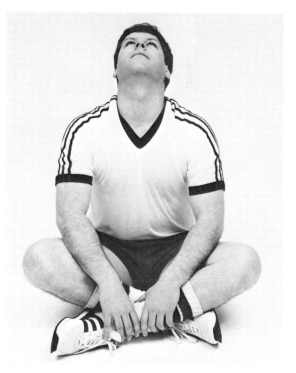

Now turn your head to the left without moving any other part of the body. Then bring your head back to center and turn as far as you can to the right. Repeat the side-to-side stretches four more times.

Next, bring your left ear to your left shoulder without dropping or raising either shoulder. Bring your head back to center and then try to touch your right ear to your right shoulder. Repeat four more times. While doing neck rolls, it is important not to overstrain. Just move your neck to a point where you are getting a good stretch but not over-reaching your muscles' abilities. Do not baby yourself, but do not overextend yourself, either.

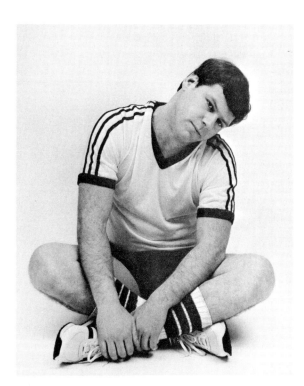 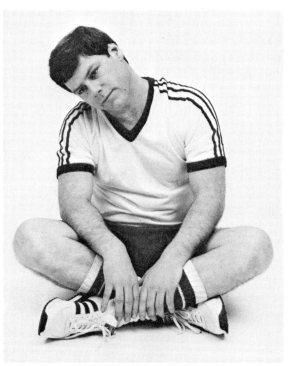

Now do some 360 degree neck rolls. First go clockwise for five slow circles; then go counterclockwise for five more rounds. Touch your chin to your chest and then roll your right ear to your right shoulder; then push your head all the way back, touch the left ear to your left shoulder, and then go back around all over again. After you have completed the full neck rolls, check to see whether there is any tension of tightness and then roll your neck back and forth in the problem areas.

Neck rolls, of course, may be done at any time during the day. Executives who find themselves reading or otherwise hunched over a desk all day often store a great deal of tension in the back of the neck. A daily program of neck rolls can help ease most of that tension as well as make the neck muscles more flexible.

Relax for a minute or two after you have finished the neck rolls. Breathe deeply and concentrate once again on relaxing.

Eye Exercises The eye exercises are next. These exercises stretch the eye muscles in a manner similar to the way neck rolls stretch the neck muscles. Executive Health Examiners knows from experience that eye exercises can relieve eyestrain problems.

Not too long ago one of our clients, a 44-year-old aeronautical engineer, found to his consternation that his right eyelid was twitching uncontrollably. He was able to stop the twitching by holding his eye wide open with his fingers, but the twitching kept coming back. Even though it was a minor problem, it was an irritating one.

The engineer consulted his eye doctor, who said there was nothing he could do. The doctor said the executive was suffering from eyestrain and suggested that he cut back on reading. When the engineer mentioned the problem to EHE doctors during a routine checkup, we suggested yoga eye exercises. The man reported that within 2 weeks after he began 5-day-a week eye exercises, the twitching went away. About a year later the engineer went on a 2-week vacation overseas. Although he did most of his regular exercises on

Eye exercises can relieve eye-strain problems.

vacation, he neglected the eye exercises. Sure enough, within a week after he returned to his job, the twitching began again. He immediately began doing the eye exercises again, and the problem disappeared within 2 weeks.

Yoga eye exercises go like this: In a comfortable cross-legged sitting position, open your eyes and without moving your head, look toward the ceiling and then to the floor. Do this ten times and then close your eyes for a few seconds. Then look to the right as far as possible without overstraining; then look to the left. Close the eyes again after ten rounds of the side-to-side stretches. When you open your eyes, look as far as you can to the upper right and then shift to the lower left. Repeat ten times. Next, look to the upper left and back to the lower right. After ten rounds, do five slow clockwise circles followed by five counterclockwise ones. Then close your eyes and rub your palms together vigorously until you feel them getting warm. Immediately cup your palms over your closed eyes without pressing the palms against the eyes, and you will feel the warmth seep in.

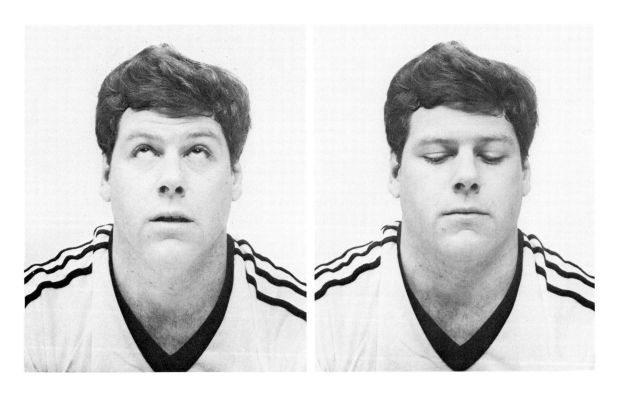

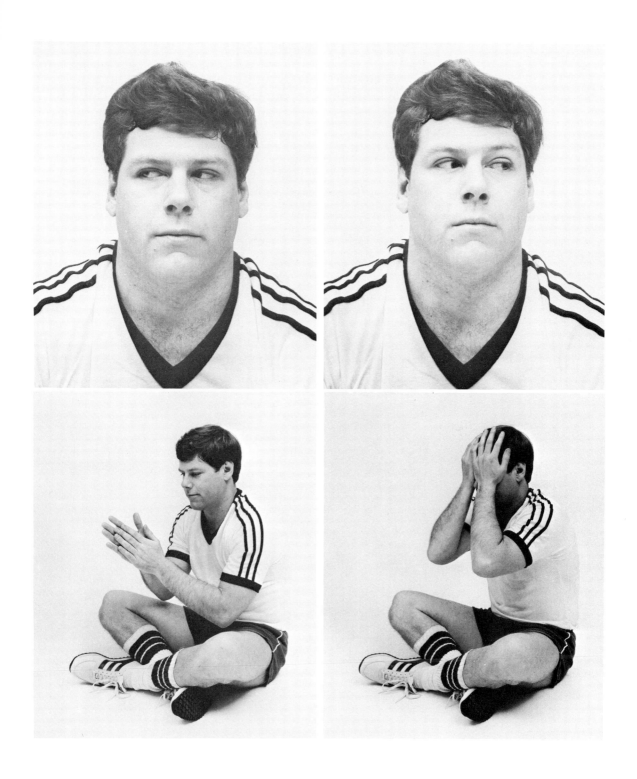

Salute to the Sun

Relax for a minute or two and then stand up and do the sun salutation. See our step-by-step instructions for this all-inclusive warmup. Try to do four, six, or eight rounds. If you feel up to it, when you are in the pushup position, go ahead and do three or four pushups.

1. Stand straight with your feet together. Hold the palms of your hands together with your fingers pointing upward.

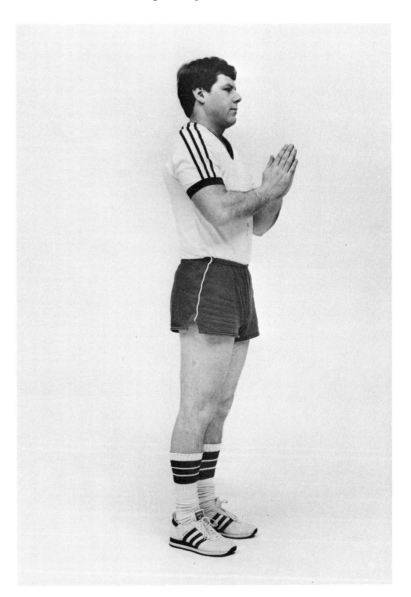

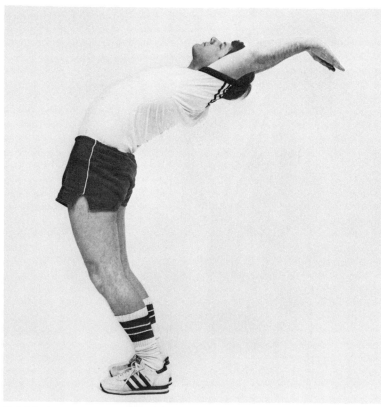

2. Lock your thumbs together and lift your arms over your head while keeping them close beside your ears. Keep your feet planted firmly on the floor, and bend backward, looking up at your hands.

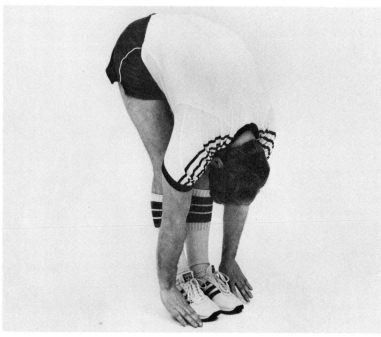

3. With your head between your arms, bend forward with your knees straight, and place the palms of your hands flat on the floor on either side of your feet. Try to have your face touch your knees.

4. *Extend your left leg back with your left knee touching the floor. Keep your right foot between your hands, and make your right knee touch your chest. Look upward.*

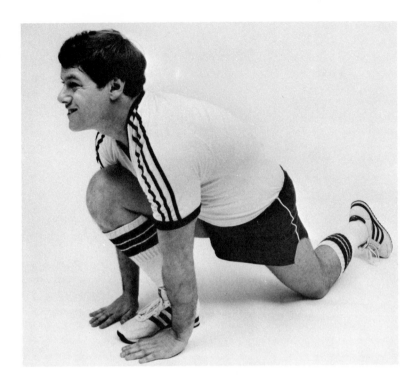

5. *Take your right leg back so that your right foot is beside your left foot and your body forms an arch. Your head should be between your arms, and you should be looking at your feet. Your heels should stay on the floor.*

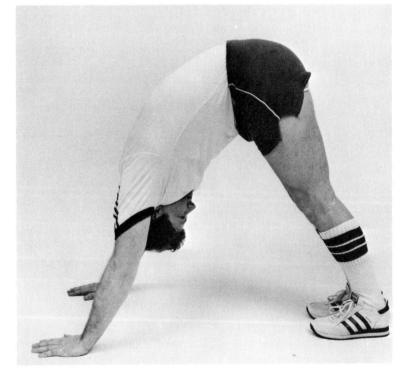

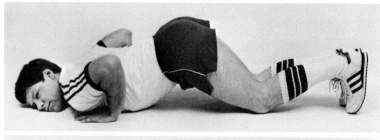

6. Lower your knees down to the floor, then your chest, then your chin. Your pelvis should be a few inches off the floor, and the palms of your hands under your shoulders.

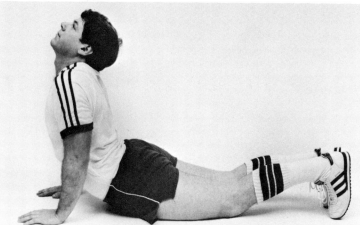

7. Lower your pelvis to the floor and raise your chest, neck, and head, and look upward. Keep your elbows slightly bent, close beside your body. Your weight in this position will rest on your back.

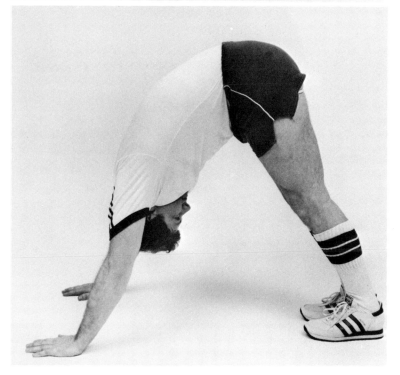

8. In one movement, lower your head between your arms, with your heels on the floor and your body arched.

9. Look upward. Move your left leg forward between your hands, with your left knee touching your chest. Your right leg should be extended back, with your right knee on the floor.

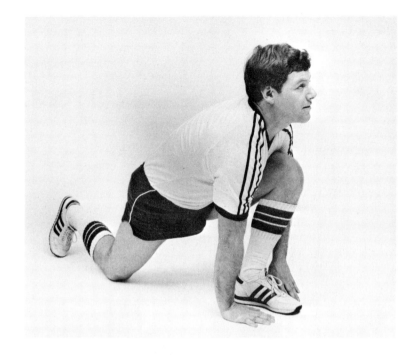

10. Move your right leg forward and straighten your knees. Put the palms of your hands flat on the floor on either side of your feet. Try to make your face touch your knees.

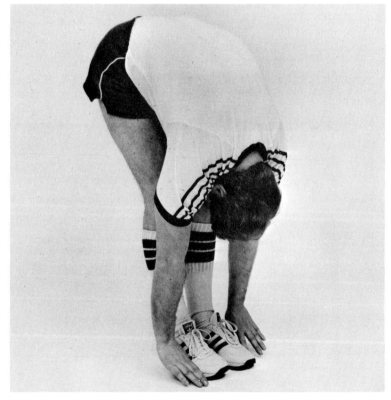

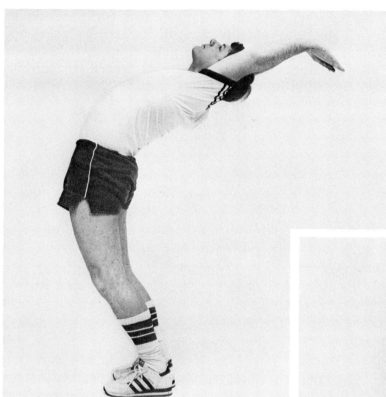

11. Keep your arms beside your body, and stretch upward and backward, looking at your hands.

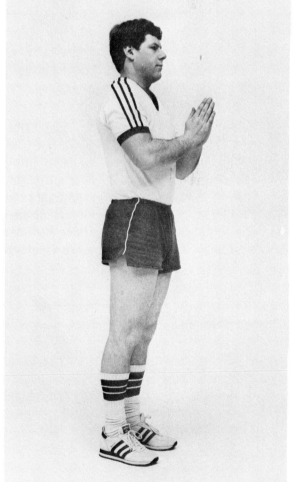

12. Stand straight, lower your arms, and bring your palms together.

After the sun salutation, lie on your back with your feet 18 inches apart and your arms away from your sides, palms up. This is the corpse, or relaxation, pose. Begin a series of deep breaths, roll your head from side to side, and shake out your legs and arms. Rest for at least 3 minutes.

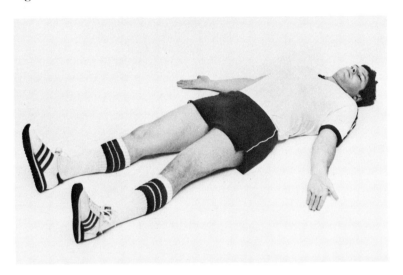

Leg Lifts The next exercises are the leg lifts. Try to keep your body relaxed as you do them. Do not tense up the face, neck, or shoulders. With your heels pointed toward the ceiling and your toes pointed toward your head, slowly lift the right leg to a count of 5. Keep the left leg straight and on the floor. Inhale as you raise the right leg to 90 degrees; then exhale and allow the leg to return slowly to the floor. Do the same with the left leg.

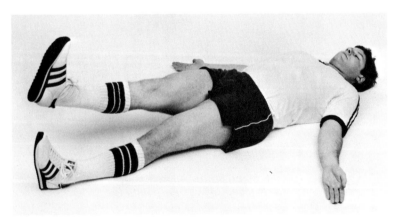

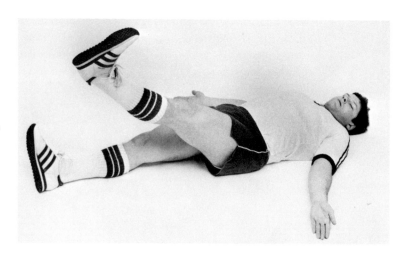

On the third or fourth round, flex your ankles while the legs are up off the ground. For the final round, reach up and grab your right leg with your hands and slowly pull it gently toward you as you raise your forehead to your knee. Repeat with the left leg. Do not forget to continue breathing deeply at all times.

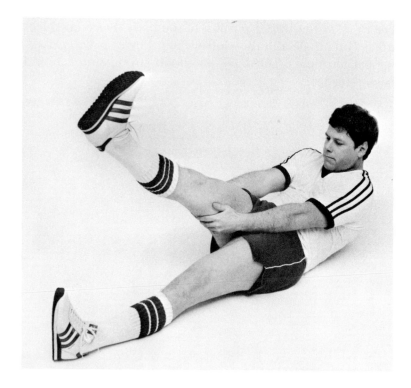

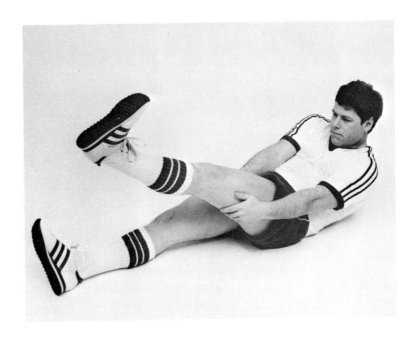

Now try double leg lifts. Keep your heels pointed to the ceiling and your toes pointed toward your head and remember to relax the upper portion of the body. Raise both legs up as you inhale and then lower them slowly as you exhale. Repeat ten times. These leg lifts build strong stomach and back muscles.

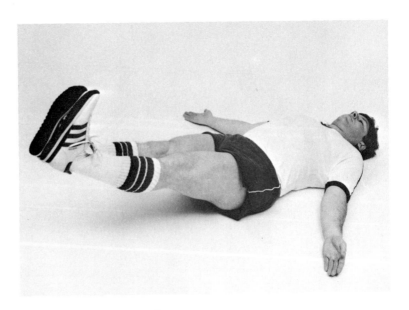

Shoulder Stands After the leg lifts, lie back down and breathe deeply for 3 to 5 minutes. Now you are ready for the first yoga posture, the shoulder stand. Place your hands, palms down, alongside your body. Raise your legs to 90 degrees and then roll your trunk into a vertical position. Slide your hands along your back for support. The back of your neck should be flat on the floor; your chin should be pressed into your chest. Breathe deeply and relax as you settle into the posture. It will feel very awkward the first few times, but try to hold the shoulder stand for at least 1 minute.

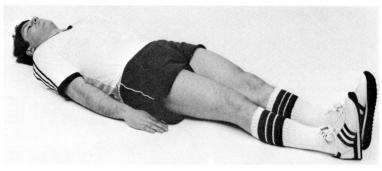

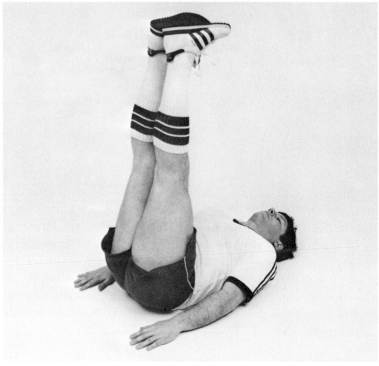

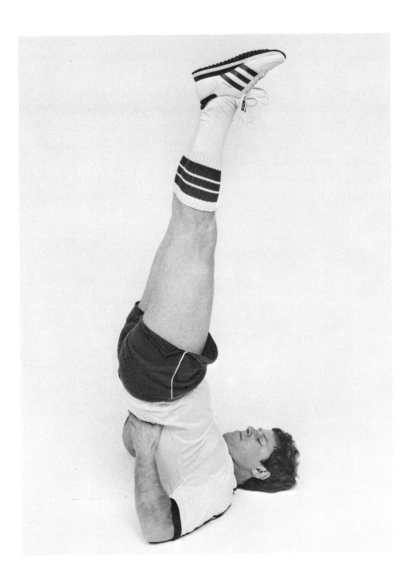

After several weeks' practice you should progress to 3 minutes; the goal is 10 minutes. The shoulder stand helps strengthen the back muscles and brings flexibility to the legs.

It's important to roll out of the shoulder stand very slowly, keeping control at all times. Do not unroll too quickly and do not let your head rise off the floor as you roll down. After the shoulder stand, immediately lie down again in the relaxation position, roll your head from side to side, and breathe deeply.

The Fish Pose The complementary posture to the shoulder stand is the fish pose. In this pose, bend the neck in the opposite direction from what it was in in the shoulder stand. Begin by placing your palms under your thighs; then arch your back and support yourself with your elbows. Try to put the crown of your head on the floor. Most of your weight should be supported by the elbows, not the head. Breathe deeply in this position but be alert to dizziness. If you feel dizzy, slowly come down and take a few breaths before trying the pose again. Hold the position as long as you can. The ideal is to hold it for about half the time you held the shoulder stand.

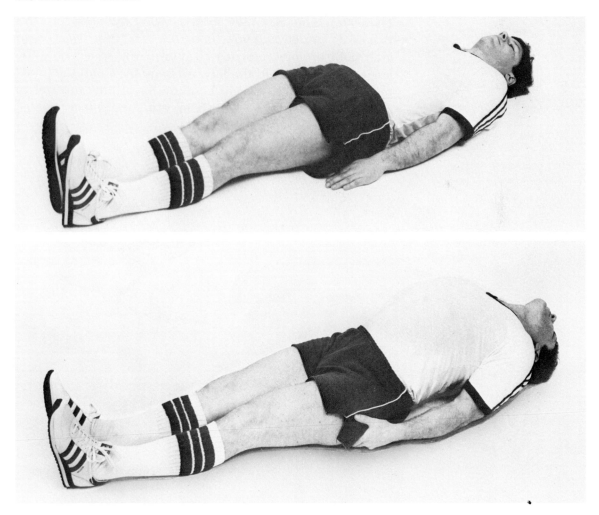

Slowly unwind and take several deep breaths. Roll your head from side to side. Bounce your legs up and down. Then to relax the neck, cup your hands behind your head and, using only your arms, pull the head forward toward the chest. Be very careful and do not overstrain. Put your head back on the floor and relax.

Forward-Bending Exercises The next set of postures are the forward-bending exercises. Begin on your back in the relaxation pose. Stretch your arms over your head and give your entire body a good long stretch. Relax and stretch again. This time stretch your arms over your head and then slowly sit up with your hands remaining over your head. Then stretch out again toward the ceiling and bend forward. Exhale as you stretch your body out over your legs. Try to grab hold of your toes. It's all right if you reach only the ankles or knees. Hold the forward bend for about a minute, remembering as always to continue breathing and not to strain overly hard. As you exhale, you should feel yourself sinking a bit lower.

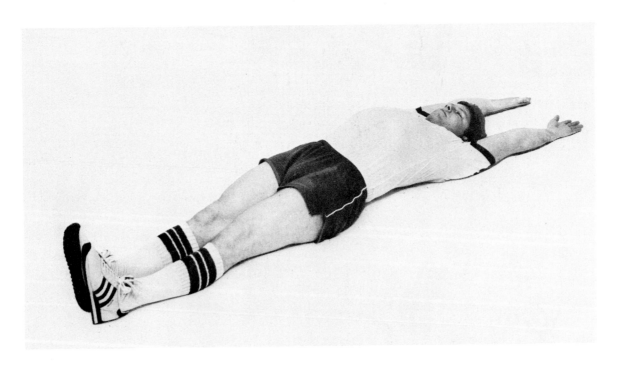

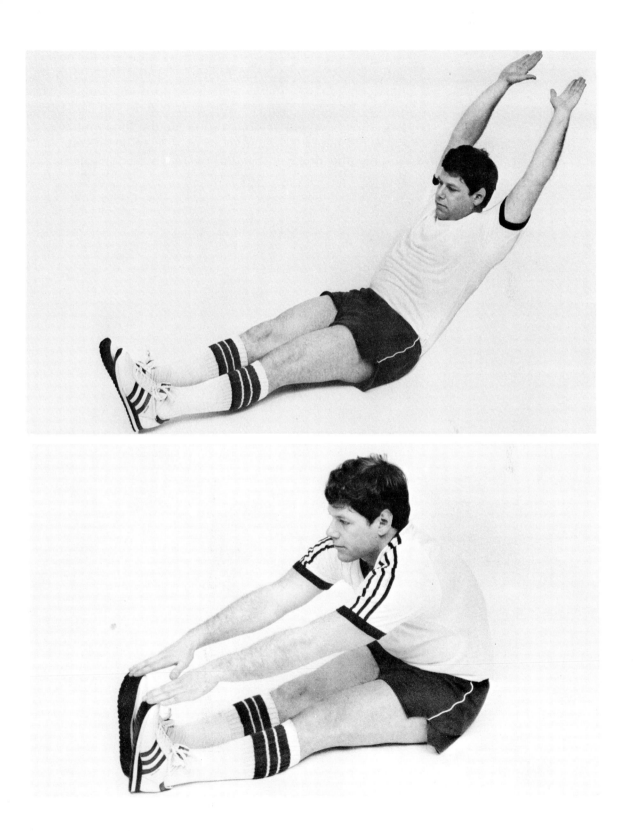

Raise yourself slowly, stretching again toward the ceiling, and then drop your arms behind you and move into the next position, the inclined plane. Supporting yourself with your arms, slowly raise your torso as high as you can, trying to get the body into a straight line. Hold it for about 20 seconds and then lower yourself slowly. Then lie on your back and breathe. Roll your head from side to side; shake out any tension in your arms and legs.

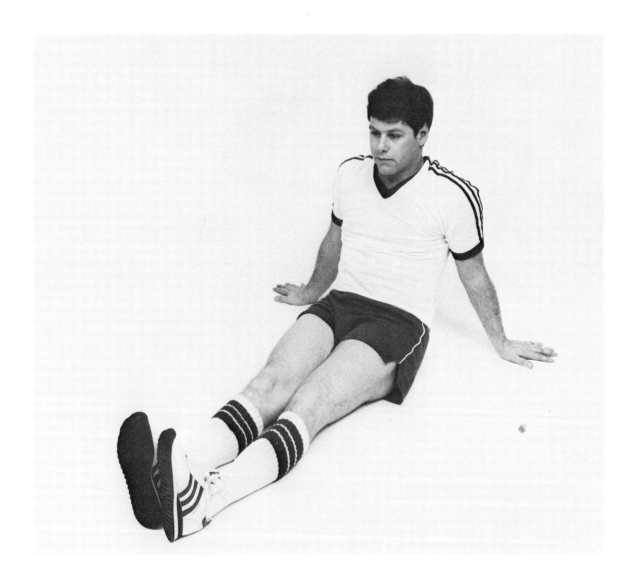

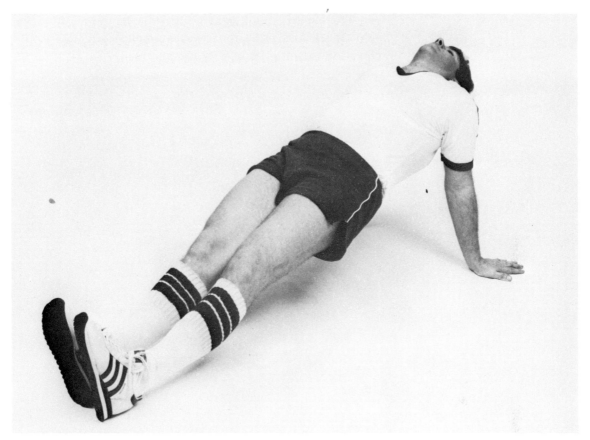

Backward-Bending Poses Complementing the forward bends, naturally enough, are the backward-bending poses. There are three basic backward bends: the cobra, the locust, and the bow. If you have time, try each one. If not, choose one that suits you best.

Roll over on your stomach in preparation for the back-bending poses. To relax on your stomach, make a pillow with your hands and rest one cheek on your top hand. Then touch your big toes and let your feet fall out to the sides. Take a few deep breaths.

Now try the cobra. Put your legs together with the toes pointed down. Put your palms under your shoulders and your forehead on the floor. Keeping your legs close together, slide slowly up into position, brushing your forehead, nose, and chin along the floor. Bring your head up, look toward the ceiling, and push with your hands. Slowly come up until your elbows are about halfway bent. Hold the position for about 20 seconds and then lower yourself slowly back to the relaxation position. Repeat twice more.

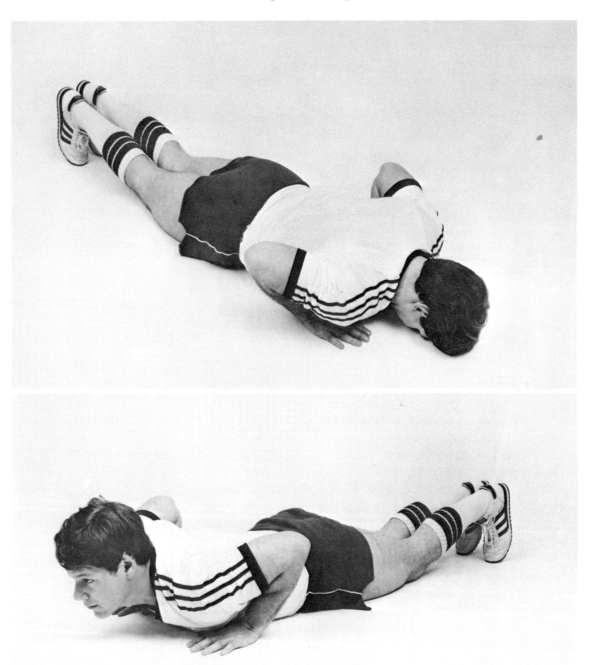

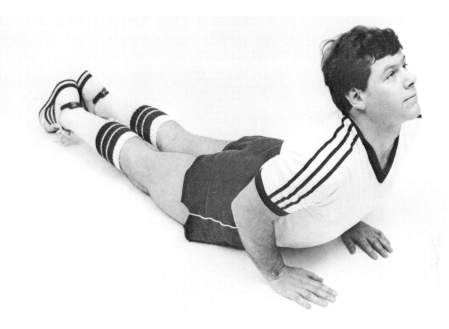

The locust is next, and it's not easy. Put your chin on the floor and bring your arms along your sides, palms down. Keeping your chin on the floor, inhale and lift the left leg up as high as it will go. Exhale and lower the leg slowly.

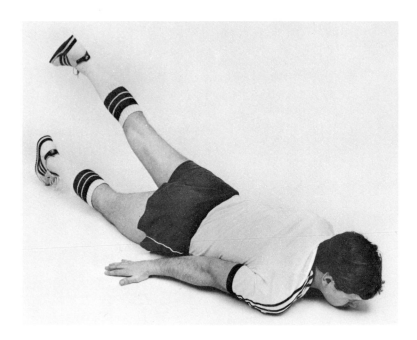

Then try the right leg. After a few single lifts with each leg, put your arms under your body, make fists with your hands, and try the full locust. Inhale deeply and lift both legs as high as you can. Try to hold them up in the air for 10 seconds and then relax.

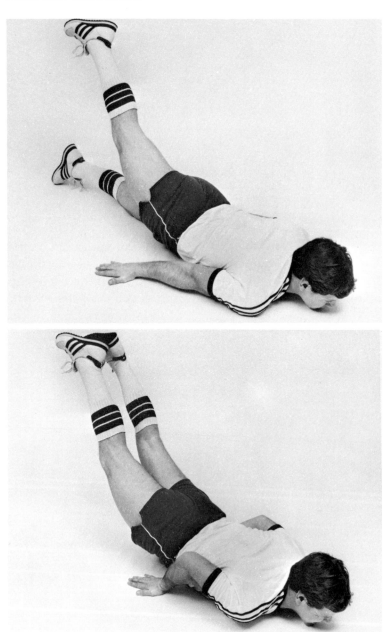

For the bow, place your forehead on the floor and reach back and grab your ankles. Then inhale and slowly lift your head, chest, and thighs; at the same time, arch your back and lift your legs. Balance on your stomach for about 5 seconds, exhale slowly, and let your head go back to the floor while you are holding on to your ankles. Try the bow again, but this time once you pull yourself up, rock back and forth six times. Then you can collapse into the relaxation position.

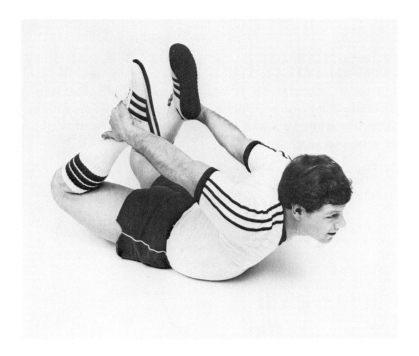

The counterpose to the back-bending positions is the child's pose. To get there from the relaxation pose, place your hands under your shoulders, come up on your knees, and sit up. Then sit back on your heels and put your forehead to the floor. Let the backs of your arms fall limply to the floor at your sides. Hold this position for at least a minute. It's very relaxing.

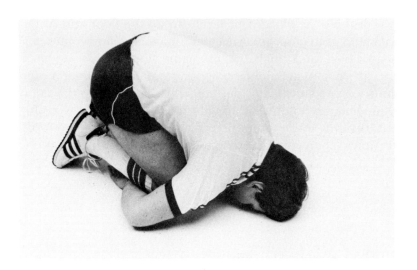

The Spinal Twist Next, sit up on your ankles and then shift your body to the right of your legs for the spinal twist, the final yoga position. This is a pretzel-like twist that helps align your spine. At first it is very uncomfortable and hard to get into, but work on it.

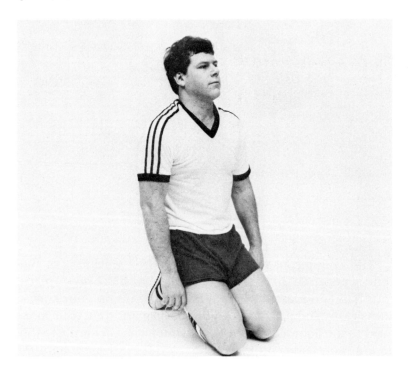

Sitting to the right of your legs, put the left leg over the right knee with the sole flat on the floor. Your left knee should be close to your chest. Then slowly twist your body to the left and raise your right arm above your head. Reach down and grab the left ankle with the right arm on the outside of your left leg. Twist your shoulders and head toward the left. Support yourself with your left hand on the floor behind your back. Hold the pose for 30 seconds. Release and twist in the opposite direction. Photos of the spinal twist are in clockwise order.

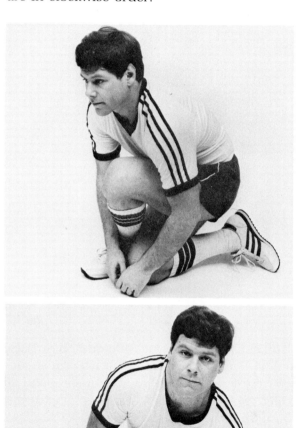

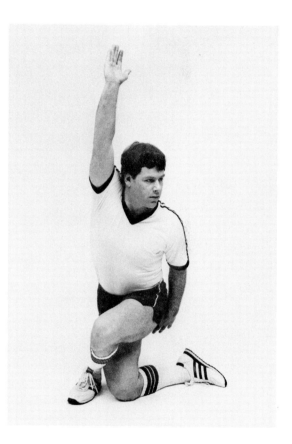

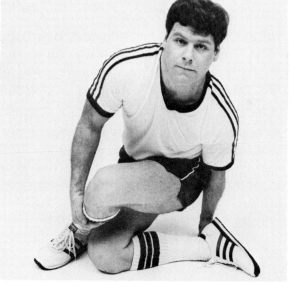

After the spinal twist you are ready for the final easy stretches. Stand up slowly. Stretch your arms to the ceiling and then let them fall loosely to the ground in front of you.

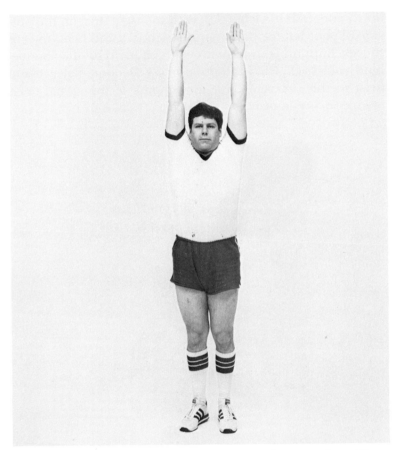

Repeat several times. Then do some side stretches. Place your feet a shoulder length apart, with your left arm at your left side and your right arm against your right ear. Bend all the way to the left. Then come back to center, change arms, and bend to the right. Repeat several times.

The Final Relaxation The last thing in your yoga routine is one of the most important, the final relaxation, which should last at least 5 minutes. You simply get into the relaxation position on your back with your legs 18 inches apart, your arms out from your sides, palms up, and your eyes closed. Roll your head from side to side several times.

Stretch your legs and arms and then relax them. Breathe deeply. Take six to eight deep diaphragmatic breaths. Spend the next 5 minutes keeping absolutely still, concentrating only on your breath.

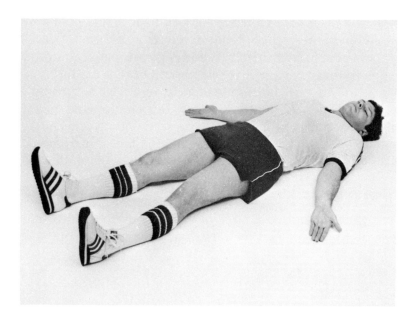

Then you are finished. Sit up slowly with your eyes closed and stay in a comfortable cross-legged position for a few seconds; then slowly open your eyes. You should be totally relaxed, stretched out, flexible, and refreshed.

Slowly open your eyes. You should be totally relaxed, stretched, flexible, and refreshed.

Suggestions for Warmup and Cooling-Down Exercises

It's best to work on stretching primarily in the warmup period for aerobics and on strength-building primarily in the cooling-down period, but you can mix the two in any way that suits you so long as you get 10 to 15 minutes of both stretching and strength building in each exercise session.

Walkers, runners, cyclists, and rope skippers can do the same warmup and cooling-down routines. The warmup can consist of six to eight rounds of the twelve-part yoga routine called the sun salutation, an exercise that stretches nearly all the muscles in the body. Or you can choose any combination of stretches that focus on the lower extremities. These include:

Standing leg stretches

You put one foot on a table or chair about 3 feet in height, extend your leg, lean forward, and try to touch your toes

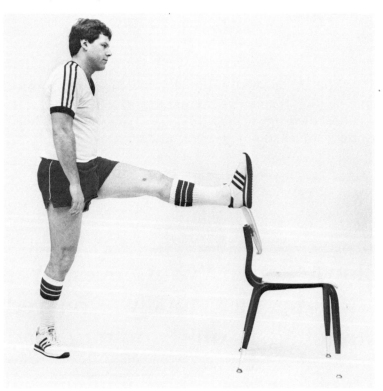

with your fingertips. This is extremely good for stretching the hamstring muscles. All you have to do is stretch each leg for about 15 to 20 seconds two or three times.

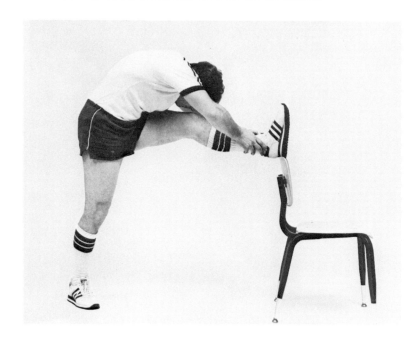

Achilles tendon and calf muscle stretches

You stand 2 to 3 feet from a wall and lean forward until your palms touch it. Then you step backward, and as your weight is supported by your hands and you remain flat-footed, the calf muscles and Achilles tendons stretch out. Do this five to ten times, holding each stretch for about 15 seconds.

The worst thing you can do right after working out is to go into a steam room, sauna, or hot shower.

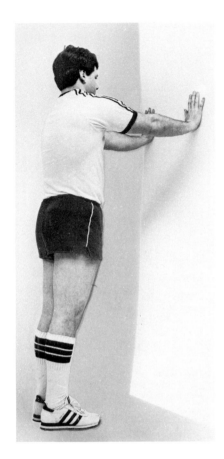
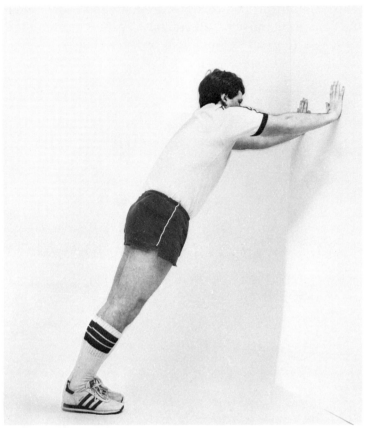

You can also try neck rolls, side stretches, and other upper-body limbering-up exercises. If you want to add calisthenics to the routine, try pushups and situps.

After you have cooled down by pedaling your bike slowly, slowing your run to a walk, or slowing your walk to a crawl, try some additional cooling down with situps, pushups, chinups (if a bar is available), and light stretching. Start these exercises in groups of six at a time; then stop, stretch out a little, and continue with another six situps, pull-ups, or whatever calisthenics you choose. After you get used to the routine and it becomes easy (this should take from 4 to 6 weeks), try increasing the sets of calisthenics exercises to ten each.

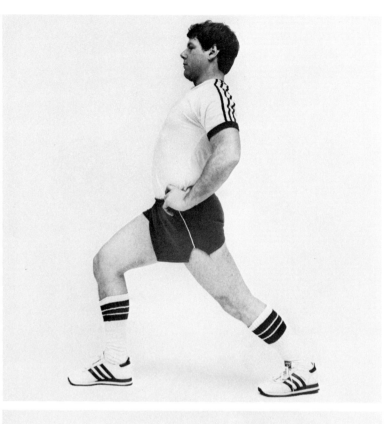

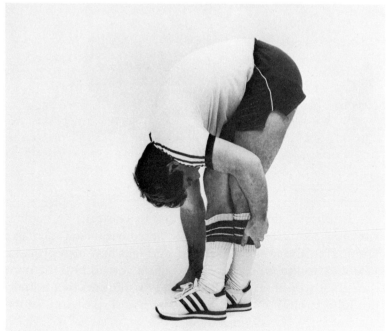

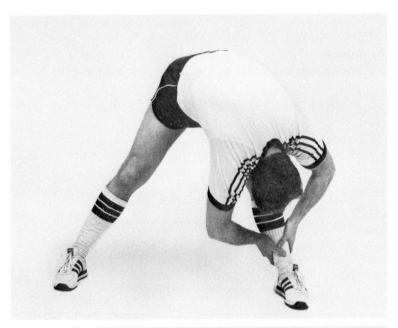

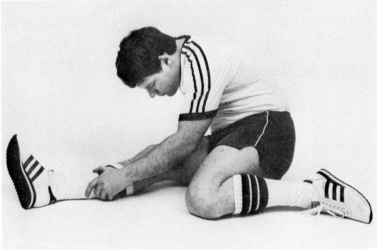

Swimmers do not need elaborate warmup or cooling-down sessions, because the aerobic activity itself increases strength in the arms, shoulders, and legs and also provides flexibility to the muscle groups. Before you go into the pool, though, it would not hurt to take a few minutes to gradually but fully stretch out your body. The twelve-part sun salutation will suffice, but you can also do any combination of stretches that gets the neck, shoulders, arms, trunk, and legs in motion.

Your first lap or two in the water also can serve as warmup time, just as the last few laps can count as cooling-down time. Just to make sure, you might want to take a few minutes to walk back and forth in the shallow end of the pool before you finish in the water. After you get out of the pool, spend a few minutes doing calisthenics. Those who swim in athletic clubs have equipment and space on hand to do situps, pushups, pullups, other calisthenics, and weight training.

If you think the cooling-down period is not necessary, remember these words of Dr. Cooper:

> The worst thing you can do right after a workout is to go into a steam room, a sauna, or a hot shower. Also, don't go sit down in your car, especially after a winter run. . . . When you combine a sudden stop of activity with a sudden decrease in warmth, the blood pools and the surface capillary vessels dilate, keeping an even greater percentage of blood away from the heart. So taper off gradually. You should take at least as long to cool down as you did to warm up. . . .

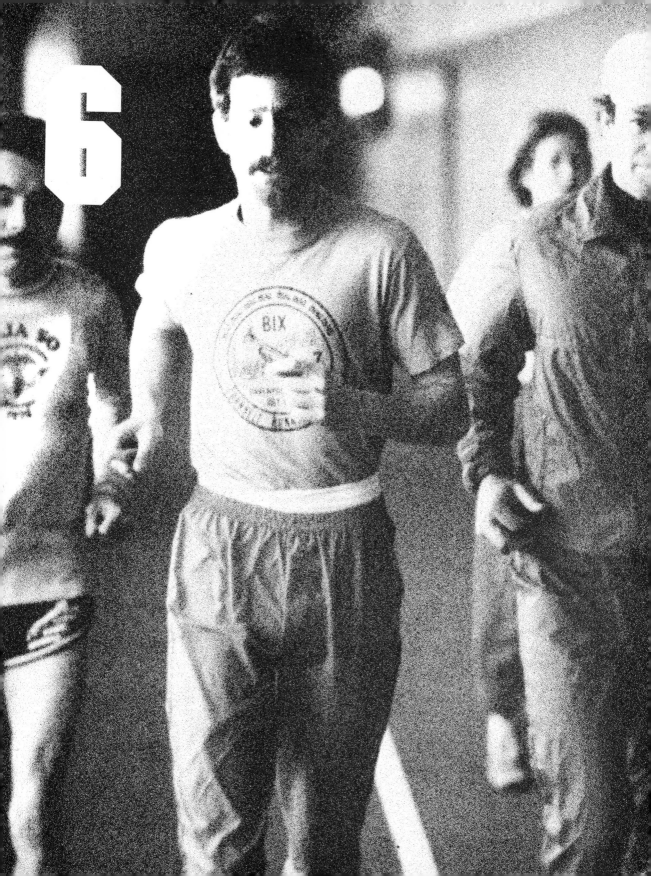

EXERCISE AT WORK

The best way to fit an exercise regimen into your daily schedule is to exercise at the office. Does this sound funny? It should not.

Hundreds of employers have now installed on-the-premise exercise facilities, including some of the nation's largest corporations, such as Exxon, General Foods, Kimberly-Clark, Firestone, Johnson&Johnson, Prudential Insurance, and Pepsico; the list also includes smaller firms such as local banks, government offices, and various other types of businesses.

According to the American Association of Fitness Directors in Business and Industry, more than 500 companies employ full-time directors to run company-sponsored fitness facilities; tens of thousands of other business organizations have some sort of organized recreation programs. The association itself, which had only 25 members when it was formed in 1974, achieved a membership of about 1800 by 1981.

Helping Employees Stay Healthy

The main reason corporations set up in-house fitness centers, of course, is to help employees stay fit, but employers also have another, less altruistic, reason. Richard O. Keelor of the President's Council on Physical Fitness and Sports says that:

> The simple truth is that fitness pays. In boardrooms and executive suites throughout the country, top management is recognizing physical fitness as a prudent investment in the health, vigor, morale, and longevity of the men and women who are the company's most valuable asset. By preventing heart attacks, disabilities, and premature retirements, fitness saves money. For the employee, half an hour's vigorous exercise can be a refreshing, needed respite from the stress and occasional tedium of work.

Doctors say that the prime cause of most back pain is lack of exercise of the back muscles.

Although no one knows the exact figures, the President's Council estimates that premature deaths cost American industry 132 million lost workdays and about $25 billion a year. There are also billions more dollars lost as a result of lowered productivity from sickness and other disabilities. Heart disease, the nation's number one killer, accounts for 52 million lost workdays each year. Back pain, which afflicts about 75 million adults, costs industry $1 billion a year in lowered productivity and $250 million annually in worker's compensation according to the National Safety Council. Doctors say that the prime cause of most back pain is lack of exercise of the back muscles. Finally, the American Heart Association reports that industry pays about $700 million a year just to recruit replacements for executives killed by premature heart attacks.

A Look at Some Different Programs

There are many types of employee fitness programs, ranging from modest, company-sponsored exercise classes at local YMCAs to highly structured, medically supervised, individualized programs undertaken at multimillion-dollar in-house exercise facilities.

The Weyerhaeuser Company's employee fitness program, begun in 1972, is set up as a nonprofit organization jointly sponsored by the company and its employees. The company has installed fitness facilities at three of its locations in Tacoma, Washington, where a director and two full-time staff members supervise the activities of 750 employees. The employees pay about $140 a year for use of the facilities, and the company picks up the cost of equipment and also pays the water, electric, and heating bills.

Weyerhaeuser has an exercise testing laboratory where employees are given a battery of tests including measurements of cardiovascular capacity, muscular strength, and flexibility. After the evaluation, each employee is put on an individual exercise program. The fitness centers have running treadmills, weight equipment, rowing machines, and outdoor jogging and bicycle trails, and there are also handball, racketball, volleyball, and basketball courts. Weyerhaeuser's fitness program also includes screening for hypertension and programs in nutrition, cardiopulmonary resuscitation, and stress management.

The Kimberly-Clark Corporation of Neenah, Wisconsin, has spent $2.5 million on its employee fitness program since the program began in October 1977. The company also conducts programs on nutrition, mental stress, and alcohol and drug abuse in a related health management program. Kimberly-Clark has about two dozen full- and part-time people running its fitness program, which is open to all employees. There are two doctors, including the director, Robert E. Dedmon, M.D., an internist, seven registered nurses, and exercise instructors.

The company's fitness complex includes a 100-meter indoor running track, an Olympic-size swimming pool, an exercise room, a sauna, a whirlpool, and the usual locker room facilities. Extensive medical tests are conducted before employees enter the program, and the testing continues while they are exercising. "Kimberly-Clark has a substantial investment in its employees," said Darwin E. Smith, chairman and chief executive officer. "To us, it is simply good business sense to keep them feeling well, which not only keeps them on the job but even helps them do a better job."[1]

Company fitness programs provide adequate exercise opportunities and close monitoring by trained professionals.

[1] Jack Martin, "The New Business Boom—Employee Fitness," *Nation's Business*, February 1978, p. 68.

Rockwell International Corporation has one of the most elaborate employee fitness centers in the country. The corporation has built several recreational facilities for employees, including a 16-acre site in El Segundo, California, which consists of a gymnasium, rifle range, tennis courts, and lighted softball diamonds.

Other company fitness programs are not as extensive or costly as Rockwell International's or Kimberly-Clark's, but they still provide adequate exercise opportunities and close monitoring by trained medical and exercise professionals. Exxon has a thirty-ninth-floor fitness center in New York City in which potential participants are screened with a complete medical examination, often including a stress test, before embarking on individualized exercise regimens. Johns Manville's $17,000 gymnasium in its Denver offices has a similar program. The Canadian firm of James Richardson and Sons has an employee fitness area, complete with running track, on the thirty-fourth floor of its office building in Winnipeg. Northern Natural Gas in Omaha took over a decaying YMCA and turned it into a company fitness center complete with swimming pool, gym, handball, racketball, and squash courts, exercise and weight rooms, and an indoor track.

THE CONCEPT OF EMPLOYEE FITNESS

In 1974, when the American Association of Fitness Directors in Business and Industry (AAFDBI) was formed, the concept of employee fitness facilities was not very well known. Since then, the rapid growth of AAFDBI has mirrored the expansion of company-sponsored, professionally run employee fitness centers.

AAFDBI had barely three dozen members in 1974. It now has some 1500 members, including about 400 professionals employed by companies or organizations as fitness directors, supervisors, coordinators, or instructors of physical fitness programs operated by firms for their employees.

AAFDBI, an affiliate of the President's Council on Physical Fitness and Sports, is in business to support and assist employers in developing physical fitness programs. The organization serves as a clearinghouse for information and services pertaining to physical fitness programs. Among other things, the association maintains a list of recommended qualifications and professional standards for fitness directors and other professional personnel in business and industry.

The mailing address is:
Room 3030
400 6th St. S.W.
Washington, DC 20201
Phone: (202) 755-7478

Leader in the Field: Pepsico

Pepsico has had employee fitness programs for two decades. As one of the leaders in programs for employee fitness, Pepsico has two basic programs: one for executives and one for all other employees.

The Pepsico executives fitness program is "based on a cost-effective model," says director Dennis Colacino. "By cost-effective, I mean preventing a key person from dying prematurely or becoming ill. We do rigorous screening for disease and cardiac stress testing to detect advanced coronary problems." Pepsico executives must either complete a physical examination by a company physician or have a letter from a personal doctor before entering the program. In addition, the executive must take a cardiac stress test as well as a "battery of pulmonary and anthropometric measurements" before beginning an exercise program.[2]

After 6 months the executive is retested and then is tested again annually. If there is any sort of cardiovascular problem, Pepsico has a special "high-risk intervention program" in which the executive is monitored closely at all times by trained medical personnel.

Among the other benefits afforded by employee fitness programs is the boost they give to company morale. As Colacino puts it: "One outcome at Pepsico is that the program, including all the recreational and fitness activities, tends to make a large company seem smaller. People get to know each other and that's a good thing." As magazine publisher Malcolm Forbes, a strong advocate of employee fitness programs, says, such activities "give the whole firm a sense of team spirit."[3]

How to Get Your Company to Become More Fitness-Conscious

As the President's Council on Physical Fitness and Sports and its affiliate, the American Association of Fitness Directors in Business and Industry, advise, the best way to get your company on the road toward setting up a fitness center is to gain the support of top management. Executive

---

[2] *The Physician and Sportsmedicine*, May 1980, p. 65.
[3] *Newsweek*, May 23, 1977, p. 79.

When a company president or chairman of the board regularly takes part in fitness activities, many of the firm's executives follow suit.

Health Examiners has found that enthusiasm for exercise is contagious. When a company president or chairman of the board regularly takes part in fitness activities, many of the firm's executives follow suit, and the company develops some sort of employee fitness program. The reverse is also true. When we see nonexercising top management people who are out of shape, most of their executives are often in the same poor condition.

Roy Larsen, M.D., vice president and medical director of Wausau Insurance Companies of Wausau, Wisconsin, explained how his company is a good example of this "trickle-down" theory of fitness. "The chairman of the board is a tennis enthusiast who carried his racket all over with him," Dr. Larsen said recently. "Our president is a dedicated swimmer, and the general counsel is a jogger and tennis player." Naturally, Wausau is a company with an extensive employee fitness program; as Dr. Larsen points out, "most of our top management are in good physical condition."

Keith Fogle, senior exercise physiologist for the Prudential Insurance Company of America in Newark, New Jersey, commented recently on the cooperation of top management in setting up employee exercise programs. "It is great when management personnel realize that they feel much better when they [for example] begin to lose weight," Fogle said. "Then they support this kind of program. This is important not only for the continuation of the program but also for expanding it. . . ."

Curtis S. Wilbur, scientific coordinator of Johnson&Johnson's New Brunswick, New Jersey, exercise program, agrees. "Many top management personnel realize the personal benefits from their own participation in a health promotion activity, and base their decision on setting up company fitness programs in part on their subjective experiences. They say to themselves, 'I don't care what the numbers are—I know this program has helped me.'"[4]

Starting Small and Growing from Within

Bob Glover, a fitness consultant and runner who has been involved in setting up many corporate fitness programs, suggests a reasoned approach to help start such programs. "You must realize that you can't just approach the chairman of the board with a great idea—building a running track, gym, lockers, etc.," Glover warns. "The best way to get your company involved is to start small and grow from within. As demand expands, you will be in a better position to ask for more fitness benefits."

Glover suggests four methods for "starting small and growing from within." One possibility is to form a company running club. The club should have monthly or bimonthly meetings complete with speakers and instructional advice. The idea is to attract runners of all levels from within the company and especially to encourage beginners. After the group gets going, it can sponsor group runs, preferably during the lunch hour. Getting a large group involved can help impress upon top management the need to set up an employee fitness program at the office. Glover suggests that the group's first request be installation of a shower so that the office will not be filled with sweating runners after lunchtime runs.

Another way to lobby for fitness facilities is to stage some sort of running event for employees at noon. "The spirit of competition for company running honors in such an event will be bound to attract the attention of upper management," Glover writes, "thus softening them for future expansion of fitness programs and facilities."

A third way of attracting attention is to set up a race with executives of other corporations. The local running club can help you organize such an event. One successful example is the annual series of 3.5-mile races in New York City's Central Park, in which employees from more than 600 corporations,

[4] Larsen, Fogle, and Wilbur quoted in *The Physician and Sportsmedicine*, May 1980, pp. 70–71.

trade organizations, and government agencies took part in 1981. The event, sponsored by the New York Road Runners Club and Manufacturers Hanover Trust bank, "is a showcase for company spirit as the park overflows with uniformed teams, cheerleaders, and banners," Glover writes. "The company parties go well into the night, and even though the competition for prizes is intense, the average employee participates and many more benefit by the excitement of their company's involvement."

Glover's final suggestion is to have the company's experienced runners set up clinics or classes for beginners. "By using a trained running instructor, a company can save the expense of creating its own program and staff," Glover points out.

What You Can Do on Your Own at Work

If your company does not have a fitness program, or if you do not have the time or the inclination to take part in one, there are ways to exercise on your own while at the office. You can exercise individual muscles when they tense up, or you can design your own program of exercises as preventive medicine.

There is also the option of undertaking a series of isometric exercises, most of which you can do while sitting at your desk. You can do neck rolls any time during the day to prevent tension from building in your neck muscles. To tighten your stomach muscles while sitting at your desk, suck in your stomach and hold your breath for 6 seconds. To tone your buttocks, take a deep breath and tighten your stomach and buttocks. Hold it for 6 seconds, relax, take another deep breath, and then repeat the exercise.

If your company does not have a fitness program, there are ways to exercise on your own at the office.

If you feel tension in your arms, place your hands on the arms of your chair and slowly lift yourself up a few inches. Hold yourself there for 5 seconds and then let yourself down slowly. Repeat several times.

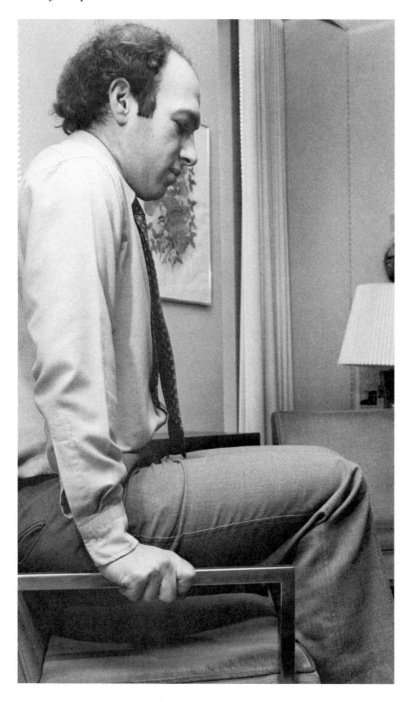

If your hands and wrists become tired from too much desk work, take time to flex them. Make tight fists, hold them for a few seconds, and then relax. Repeat several times. Let your wrists go limp and then shake your hands as if you were trying to dry them. Relax the hands and then make quick tight fists; follow this by throwing open your fingers several times. Shake out the hands again and go back to work.

If your legs are stiff from too much sitting, get up and walk around the office for a few minutes. Or stay in your chair and grab one knee with both hands. Pull the knee toward your chest. Do several rounds with each knee and finally hug both knees and pull them to your chest one last time. Hold your legs in that position for a few seconds; then

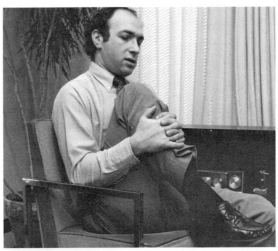

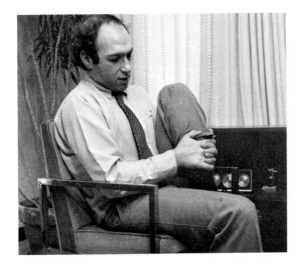

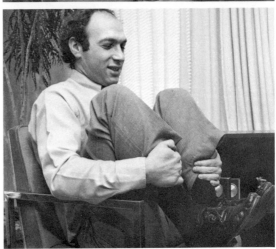

stand up and raise yourself up and down on your toes (take off your shoes if you feel like it). After you have gone up and down on your toes a half dozen times, roll back and forth on your heels for a minute or so.

While you are standing, stretch your arms a bit, lean forward, and touch your toes with your knees bent slightly. Slowly come up and stretch toward the ceiling and then back to the toes.

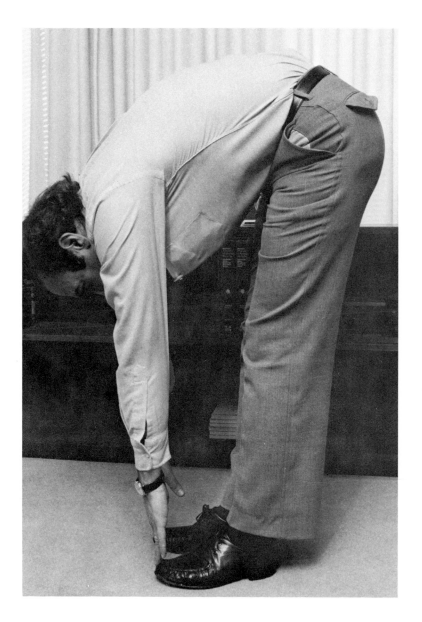
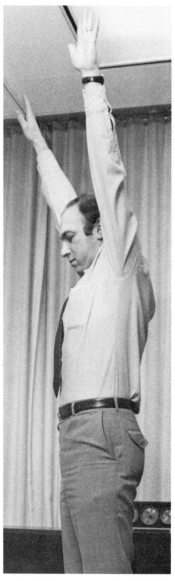

Do some knee lifts, raising each knee as high as possible and grabbing your legs with your hands and pulling the knees alternatively against your body. Be sure to keep your back straight.

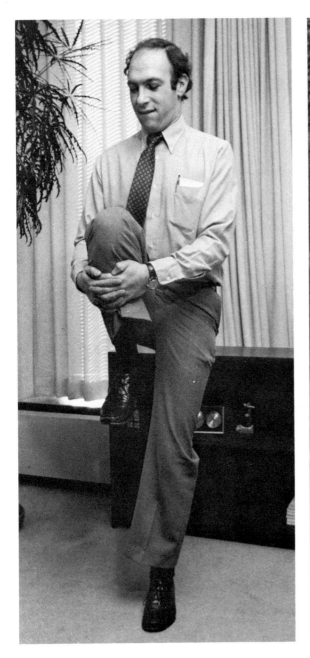 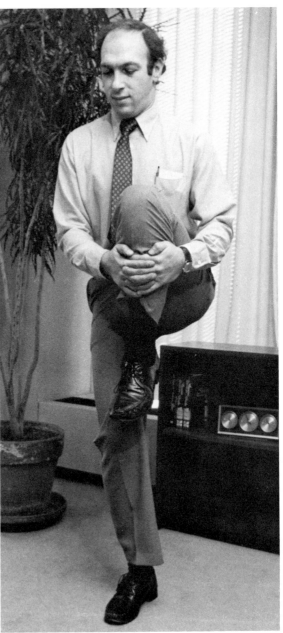

You can even lift "weights" in the office without dragging in a set of barbells. Take a book in each hand and lift them slowly over your head and back down to your sides. Repeat this several times.

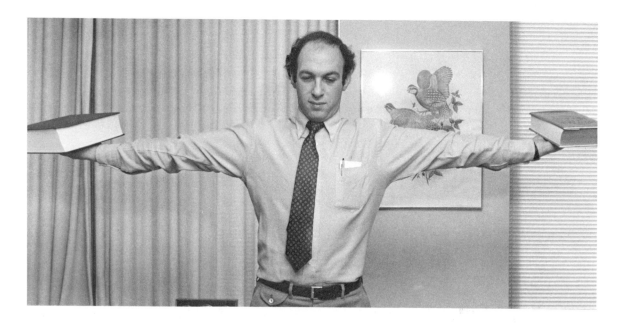

The stair climb, as we mentioned earlier, does not provide aerobic benefit, but it helps build leg muscles and keep you mentally alert at the office by getting you out from behind your desk and moving around. The way to get the most out of stair climbing at the office is to climb three flights of 9-inch steps at a 30- to 40-step-per-minute pace in 30 seconds or less. If you can handle it, take the steps two at a time. If you can do nine or ten of these 30-second workouts during the day, you will have accomplished a fruitful mini-exercise regimen.

Remember, as with any other exercise routine, you must begin your stair climbing slowly and progress gradually. This can be vigorous exercise; if you are in poor physical shape, you risk injury by dashing up the stairs without warming up properly.

There are several other precautions to take before you do stair climbing at the office. Check out the staircases to see whether the doors are unlocked. Sometimes the interior staircase doors of office buildings are locked from the inside for security purposes. Also make sure the stairways are sufficiently lighted. You should be able to see where you are going; otherwise, you risk a potentially nasty spill.

You should also check with building management to see if it's acceptable to have you running up the stairs during the workday. Some buildings do not allow this type of activity. It's also a good idea to see if you can talk a coworker or two into venturing into the stairwell with you. It's not that misery loves company, but as in any exercise routine, you get a psychological lift when you have someone to share the exercise with.

The Six Categories of Company Fitness Programs

The President's Council on Physical Fitness and Sports divides employee fitness programs into six categories. Leading the list is the complete on-site program. Such a program should be phased in over a 3- to 5-year period, mainly because it requires time to build a facility or refurbish an existing unused area. The top priority for a complete on-site program is hiring a trained, experienced health/fitness director and a support staff of fitness specialists. The American Association of Fitness Directors in Business and Industry maintains a list of trained specialists in the field; it is available to any company considering employing a health professional and may be obtained by contacting the association at 400 6th St. S.W., Washington, DC 20201.

As with any exercise routine, you must begin stair climbing slowly and progress gradually.

The President's Council recommends that fitness programs be run by the company's medical director. Companies that do not have medical directors should employ outside medical and fitness authorities to examine all employees before they begin their exercise programs.

The second recommended type of program involves a company contracting with an outside organization such as a local YMCA to direct the firm's on-site program. This is especially recommended for firms that do not have medical directors. A third option is contracting to run the program at the YMCA or another organization that has facilities and instructors. Smaller companies and branches of larger ones have used this concept with good results. The Maxwell House division of General Foods, at their plant in New Jersey, turned its employee training over to the experts and facilities at a nearby Y.

A fourth possibility is setting up share-cost programs in which the company and the employees split the expenses of the exercise program at the Y or health club. The fifth program involves setting up minimal exercise facilities for employees who are interested in fitness and want to work out at the office. This includes installing showers for those who run or bicycle to work or exercise during the lunch hour. It also includes setting up bike racks or secured bicycle rooms for those who commute by bicycle. Finally, there is the bare minimum program: an educational effort by the company to assess the health of employees and to instruct them on how to begin exercising on their own.

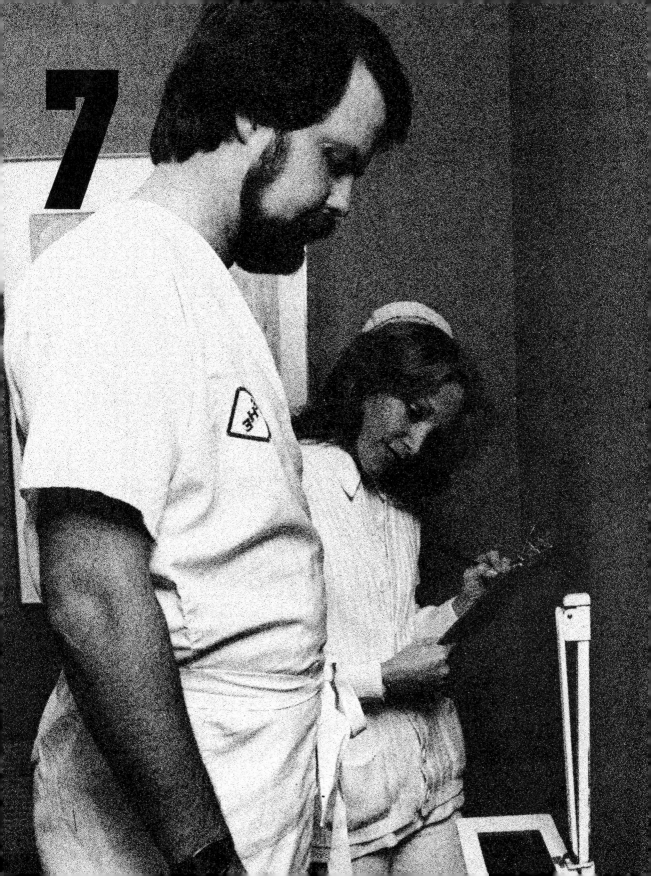

WEIGHT REDUCTION: CALORIES AND CALORIE BURNING

You probably know someone like him. He is a senior vice president of a large wholesale furniture manufacturer in the northeast, and he is always on a diet. When he first came to Executive Health Examiners, he told us he had tried the Stillman water diet, the Scarsdale diet, the Drinking Man's diet, and about a dozen others he could not even remember. He usually had great success the first few days of a new diet, he confided, having once lost 5 pounds in 3 days. Another time he dropped 7 pounds the first week. After these startling weight losses, he goes back to his normal eating patterns. Within a few months he gains all the weight back, and once again he is looking for another diet.

The experts say that this man is typical of the 80 to 90 percent of American dieters who jump from one fad diet to another in ultimately unsuccessful attempts to lose weight. Nutritionist and Tufts University president Jean Mayer calls this phenomenon "the rhythm method of girth control." George A. Bray, M.D., who edits the *International Journal of Obesity* at the University of California at Los Angeles, is one of the many experts who say that none of these diets will help you lose weight. "It seems obvious from the number of diets that have been made available and are continuing to appear, none of them provides the answer to obesity," Dr. Bray said recently.[1]

Our overweight, diet-jumping executive—as well as millions of other chronically overweight Americans who turn to one fad diet after another—has not figured out a very obvious, commonsense medical fact: Losing weight simply is a matter of arithmetic. If you consume more calories than you burn, you gain weight. If you burn more calories than you consume, you lose. The executive keeps gaining and losing weight because he only varies the amount of calories he takes in and disregards the calories he burns.

Weight Loss through Exercise

The best way to lose weight is to cut down the amount of high-caloric foods you consume every day while at the same time burning off extra calories through a balanced exercise program which emphasizes aerobics. Exercising works in two ways to burn up calories. First, during the exercise period itself the body is forced to work harder and burn extra calories. Second, studies have shown that vigorous exercise raises the basal metabolic rate (the rate at which calories are burned when the body is at rest) for as long as 15 hours after you have finished working out.

As the case of the constantly dieting furniture executive illustrates, you can lose weight by going on a drastic diet and not exercising. However, the weight loss usually con-

[1] Interview in the *New York Times*, February 24, 1981.

Losing weight is a matter of arithmetic. If you consume more calories than you burn, you gain weight. If you burn more calories than you consume, you lose weight.

sists mostly of a loss of body water, and the pounds will come back once you have returned to your normal eating patterns. If you want to lose weight and keep it off, all you have to do is burn more calories than you consume. Once you have reached your ideal weight, if you keep the amount of calories consumed and burned in balance, you will maintain that weight.

The validity of this arithmetic of weight control has been borne out in a number of medical experments. Grant Gwinup, M.D., of the University of California at Irvine, examined thirty-four chronically overweight women whose weight ranged from 134 to 218 pounds and who were 10 to 60 percent overweight. None had ever been on a truly successful diet. Dr. Gwinup decided to see whether these women could lose weight without changing their eating habits. Each subject began an exercise program that involved a brisk daily 30-minute walk. The results were astounding. The eleven women who completed the 60-week program lost an average of 22 pounds. Every woman lost weight, but none went on a diet.

Another study, conducted by Drs. W. B. Zuti and L. A. Golding of Kent State University, came up with similar results. Zuti and Golding examined the weight-reduction progress of a group of women who did enough exercise to burn 500 calories a day but did not change their eating habits. These women, some of whom were 40 pounds overweight, chose whatever exercise they wanted as long as it burned up 500 calories a day. Without altering their diets, the women lost an average of 10.6 pounds in 16 weeks.

No Quick Results

Losing weight through diet and exercise is not easy. You have to work at it, especially in the beginning. It's hard enough for overweight people to cut back on food, and it's doubly hard to stick to an exercise regimen when you are overweight and out of shape, but the physical and mental effort is worthwhile. If you follow our exercise prescription and keep an eye on your daily caloric intake, you will soon not only be losing weight, you will be looking and feeling better.

Losing weight through diet and exercise is not easy. You have to work at it, especially in the beginning.

But it will take time. You cannot lose weight quickly through exercise, because it takes a large amount of exercise to burn calories. To work off the 101 calories in just one large apple, you would have to walk for about 19 minutes, ride a bicycle for 12 minutes, swim for 9 minutes, or run for 5 minutes.

As Kenneth Cooper points out, the average person burns about 1200 calories running for 1 hour at an average pace of 6 minutes per mile.[2] That is only about half the calories an adult consumes every day. If that sounds discouraging, it should not. The idea in losing weight through diet and exercise is to work slowly but steadily. If you eat a balanced, low-calorie diet and follow an aerobic exercise program, you can lose 20 pounds or more within 6 months. All you have to do is maintain a moderate level of food intake and increase your exercise activity only slightly. Cardiologist Lenore Zohman and her colleagues have written: "If you increase your activity level only modestly, in a year you will weigh less. Certainly, if you diet as well—not crash diet, but follow a sensible and nutritious program—you will lose weight faster and enjoy good health and renewed vigor."[3]

You will lose weight gradually, but you will also lose it permanently. Not only that, you will be making permanent changes in your diet and exercise habits. This changing pattern of diet and exercise is a type of behavior modification, and in the end, behavior modification is the only answer for long-term weight control. It's a question of changing bad living habits, and you should keep in mind that habits can be

[2] *Aerobics*, p. 137.

[3] Lenore R. Zohman, et al., *The Cardiologists' Guide to Fitness and Health through Exercise* (New York: Simon and Schuster, 1979).

WORKING OFF THOSE CALORIES

Food	Calories	MINUTES OF ACTIVITY				
		Walking	Bicycling	Swimming	Running	Reclining
Apple, large	101	19	12	9	5	78
Bacon, 2 strips	96	18	12	9	5	74
Banana, small	88	17	11	8	4	68
Beans, green, 1 c.	27	5	3	2	1	21
Beer, 1 glass	114	22	14	10	6	88
Bread and butter	78	15	10	7	4	60
Cake, 2-layer, $\frac{1}{12}$	356	68	43	32	18	274
Carbonated beverage, 1 glass	106	20	13	9	5	82
Carrot, raw	42	8	5	4	2	32
Cereal, dry, $\frac{1}{2}$ c. with milk, sugar	200	38	24	18	10	154
Cheese, cottage, 1 tbsp.	27	5	3	2	1	21
Cheese, Cheddar, 1 oz.	111	21	14	10	6	85
Chicken, fried, $\frac{1}{2}$ breast	232	45	28	21	12	178
Chicken, TV dinner	542	104	66	48	28	417
Cookie, plain	15	3	2	1	1	12
Cookie, chocolate chip	51	10	6	5	3	39
Doughnut	151	29	18	13	8	116
Egg, fried	110	21	13	10	6	85
Egg, boiled	77	15	9	7	4	59
French dressing, 1 tbsp.	59	11	7	5	3	45
Halibut steak, $\frac{1}{4}$lb.	205	39	25	18	11	158
Ham, 2 slices	167	32	20	15	9	128
Ice cream, $\frac{1}{6}$ qt.	193	37	24	17	10	148
Ice cream soda	255	49	31	23	13	196
Ice milk, $\frac{1}{6}$ qt.	144	28	18	13	7	111
Gelatin, with cream	117	23	14	10	6	90
Malted milk shake	502	97	61	45	26	386
Mayonnaise, 1 tbsp.	92	18	11	8	5	71
Milk, 1 glass	166	32	20	15	9	128
Milk, skim, 1 glass	81	16	10	7	4	62
Milk shake	421	81	51	38	22	324
Orange, medium	68	13	8	6	4	52
Orange juice, 1 glass	120	23	15	11	6	92
Pancake with syrup	124	24	15	11	6	95
Peach, medium	46	9	6	4	2	35
Peas, green, $\frac{1}{2}$ c.	56	11	7	5	3	43
Pie, apple, $\frac{1}{6}$	377	73	46	34	19	290
Pie, raisin, $\frac{1}{6}$	437	84	53	39	23	336
Pizza, cheese, $\frac{1}{8}$	180	35	22	16	9	138
Pork chop, loin	314	60	38	28	16	242
Potato chips, 1 serving	108	21	13	10	6	83
Sandwiches:						
Club	590	113	72	53	30	454
Hamburger	350	67	43	31	18	269
Roast beef with gravy	430	83	52	38	22	331
Tuna fish salad	278	53	34	25	14	214
Sherbert, $\frac{1}{6}$ qt.	177	34	22	16	9	136
Shrimp, French fried	180	35	22	16	9	138
Spaghetti, 1 serving	396	76	48	35	20	305
Steak, T-bone	235	45	29	21	12	181
Strawberry shortcake	400	77	49	36	21	308

Note: Energy costs—walking for 150-lb person = 5.2 cal/min at 3.5 mph; cycling = 8.2 cal/min; swimming = 11.2 cal/min; running = 19.4 cal/min; reclining = 1.3 cal/min.

SOURCE: Adapted from F. Konishi, "Food Energy Equivalents of Various Activities," Copyright The American Dietetic Association. Reprinted by permission from the *Journal of the American Dietetic Association,* Vol. 46, 1965, pp. 186–188.

> If you eat a balanced low-calorie diet and follow an aerobic exercise program, you can lose 20 pounds or more in 6 months.

made as well as broken. It will take time, because you are trying to break habits formed over many years. Some people need professional guidance to help them change their sedentary lifestyles, but Executive Health Examiners has found that most executives who learn the facts about diet, exercise, and weight control can modify their eating habits and control their weight on their own.

Psychologists have studied the characteristics of people who have lost weight by successfully modifying their behavior on their own. Their characteristics mirror those of many successful executives. They tend to be self-disciplined, dependable, and readily willing to accept the consequences of their own behavior. They also tend to be vain.

Exercise Increases Appetite: A Myth

"I can't lose weight and exercise at the same time," a chronically overweight New Jersey account executive told EHE doctors during a recent checkup. "When I do the least bit of vigorous exercise, I'm famished afterwards. Then I eat even more than I usually do. So what's the use of exercising when I immediately eat as many calories as I burn up?"

Does exercise increase appetite? For most people, no. Dr. Mayer says the idea that exercise increases appetite is a myth that:

> seems to have incredible staying power. This may be because many people believe that an increase in physical activity always causes an increase in appetite and food intake which is at least as great in calorie replacement as the calories expended in exercise. This is not necessarily true. Actually, in a

normally active person exercise often depresses the appetite for a period of time.[4]

It is true that a well-conditioned, lean person sometimes will eat more than usual after vigorous activity, but that person has nothing to worry about. The extra exercise that caused him or her to eat more will burn up the extra calories. Some obese people, like the New Jersey advertising man, may get the urge to gorge after exercising to excess, but as Dr. Mayer and other medical authorities point out, for nearly everyone else, vigorous exercise actually *depresses* the appetite.

When you have finished a vigorous aerobic exercise session of running, walking, cycling, swimming, or jumping rope, you will not be famished. If, as Dr. Cooper recommends for dieters, you do your aerobic exercise shortly before your biggest meal of the day, you will want to eat less than you usually do. Exercise can therefore make following a diet much, much easier.

Dangers of Obesity

The dangers to health of long-term obesity are well known. Medical scientists strongly suspect that obesity is linked to heart disease, certain forms of cancer, diabetes, and stroke. A 1960 study by the Metropolitan Life Insurance Company

[4] Quoted in "Gift of Energy," p. 36.

A well-conditioned, lean person may eat more than usual after vigorous activity, but that person has nothing to worry about. The exercise that caused him or her to eat more will burn up the extra calories.

---

found that men who are 10 percent overweight run a 30 percent higher risk of early death from diabetes, heart attack, or stroke than men of normal weight. Men who are 20 percent overweight, Metropolitan Life statistics indicate, are nearly twice as likely to die prematurely. Overweight women have a higher mortality rate than women of average weight.

Determining Your Desirable Weight

There has been considerable controversy among medical experts recently over what the desirable weight for adults should be. Metropolitan Life's table of desirable weights, based on those 1960 statistics, had been the standard for two decades, but in 1981 several researchers challenged those statistics, claiming that they were based on faulty data and may be as much as 15 pounds too low.

Even as medical researchers debate what the desirable weights should be, they all agree that adult obesity presents untoward health risks—and these risks increase the longer you stay obese. Theodore Van Itallie, M.D., professor of medicine at Columbia University, summed up the prevailing medical opinion on the subject: "It's clear that we will have to be more flexible in what we think of as being obese," he said. But Van Itallie added that while optimal weights may now be thought to be slightly higher than they have been, "the dangers of obesity accelerate the further you move away from the average."[5]

EHE doctors have devised a chart that reflects what they have learned from working with executives. These figures represent the ideal weights for men and women aged 35 and over. If you are 10 to 20 percent heavier than the ideal weight for your height, you are overweight. If you are more than 20 percent over the ideal weight, you are obese.

Another way to determine whether you are overweight is to find out the proportion of your body that is muscle and the proportion that is fat. Doctors determine fat and muscle percentages in a number of ways, including immersion and

[5] Quoted in R. Lewin, "Overblown Reports Distort Obesity Risks," *Science*, January 16, 1981, Vol. 211, p. 258.

IS YOUR WEIGHT IDEAL?

Men

Height		Weight
Feet	Inches	Pounds
5	2	118
5	3	124
5	4	130
5	5	136
5	6	142
5	7	148
5	8	154
5	9	160
5	10	166
5	11	172
6	0	178
6	1	184
6	2	190
6	3	196
6	4	202
6	5	208

Women

Height		Weight
Feet	Inches	Pounds
4	10	90
4	11	95
5	0	100
5	1	105
5	2	110
5	3	115
5	4	120
5	5	125
5	6	130
5	7	135
5	8	140
5	9	145
5	10	150
5	11	155
6	0	160
6	1	165

Note: These tables represent maximum allowable weights for the average executive.

weighing under water and the use of a caliper to measure and compute skin folds. A well-conditioned man has less than 14 percent fat, a well-conditioned woman less than 20 percent. The average nonathletic man is about 18 percent fat; the average nonathletic woman, about 25 percent.

Jim Fixx suggests another way to determine whether you are carrying excessive body weight. He says that the most reliable way to find out is to take off your clothes and simply look at yourself in a mirror. If your waist is at all puffy and the skin is not stretched tight across your chest, ribs, and abdomen, you are fatter than you should be."[6]

What Type of Exercise Is Best for Weight Reduction?

You have just determined that you need to lose weight. Your next question is, What is the best exercise for weight control? Doctors say that nearly any type of exercise will help you lose weight. However, the most efficient and most beneficial exercises for weight control are the ones Executive Health Examiners recommends as the basis for the executive's overall program: aerobic exercises. Aerobic exercises are best for weight control for the same basic reasons they are best for cardiovascular conditioning. They involve constant movement of the major muscle groups, they are long in duration, and they are low in intensity. In addition, there is an extra bonus for the overweight person who follows the EHE exercise prescription. Not only will he or she lose weight permanently, but along with that weight loss will come the improvement in cardiovascular conditioning that is the basis of the executive's exercise program.

The basics of the sound diet needed to keep you from gaining weight are well known. The diet should include daily, moderate balanced amounts of foods from the three food groups: meat and dairy products, fresh vegetables and fruit, and grains, cereals, nuts, and seeds. The diet should contain little or no refined sugars or salt and should be low in highly refined and processed foods. Finally, it is important to keep a close watch on calories consumed to match

[6] James Fixx, *The Complete Book of Running* (New York: Random House, 1977).

them with the amount of calories you expend in your daily exercises.

1 *Exercises Burning up to 50 Calories*

Walk $\frac{1}{2}$ mile in 7:30 minutes
Walk/jog $\frac{1}{4}$ mile in 3 minutes
Swim 250 yards in 7:30 minutes
Cycle $1\frac{1}{2}$ miles in 9 minutes

2 *Exercises Burning 50–99 Calories*

Walk 1 mile in 15 minutes
Walk/jog $\frac{3}{4}$ mile in 9 minutes
Run $\frac{3}{4}$ mile in 6 minutes
Swim 450 yards in 15 minutes
Cycle 3 miles in 18 minutes

3 *Exercises Burning 100–149 Calories*

Walk $1\frac{1}{2}$ miles in 30 minutes
Walk/jog 1 mile in 12 minutes
Run 1 mile in 8 minutes
Swim 900 yards in 30 minutes
Cycle 3 miles in 12 minutes

4 *Exercises Burning 150–199 Calories*

Walk $2\frac{1}{2}$ miles in 50 minutes
Walk/jog $1\frac{1}{2}$ miles in 18 minutes
Run $1\frac{1}{2}$ miles in 12 minutes
Swim 1500 yards in 50 minutes
Cycle $4\frac{1}{2}$ miles in 18 minutes

5 *Exercises Burning 200–249 Calories*

Walk 3 miles in 45 minutes
Walk/jog 2 miles in 24 minutes
Run 2 miles in 16 minutes
Swim 1350 yards in 45 minutes
Cycle 6 miles in 24 minutes

AN EXERCISE SELECTOR FOR BURNING UP SPECIFIC AMOUNTS OF CALORIES

6 Exercises Burning 250–299 Calories

Walk 4 miles in 1 hour and 20 minutes
Walk/jog $2\frac{1}{4}$ miles in 27 minutes
Run $2\frac{1}{2}$ miles in 20 minutes
Swim 2400 yards in 1 hour and 20 minutes
Cycle 12 miles in 1 hour and 12 minutes

7 Exercises Burning 300–349 Calories

Walk 5 miles in 1 hour and 40 minutes
Walk/jog $2\frac{3}{4}$ miles in 39 minutes
Run 3 miles in 24 minutes
Swim 1350 yards in 24 minutes
Cycle 9 miles in 24 minutes

8 Exercises Burning 350–399 Calories

Walk $5\frac{1}{2}$ miles in 1 hour 36 minutes
Walk/jog 3 miles in 36 minutes
Run $3\frac{1}{2}$ miles in 28 minutes
Swim 1350 yards in 36 minutes
Cycle 9 miles in 36 minutes

9 Exercises Burning 400–449 Calories

Walk 6 miles in 1 hour and 45 minutes
Walk/jog $3\frac{3}{4}$ miles in 45 minutes
Run $3\frac{3}{4}$ miles in 30 minutes
Swim 1575 yards in 42 minutes
Cycle $10\frac{1}{2}$ miles in 42 minutes

10 Exercises Burning 450–500 Calories

Walk 7 miles in 2 hours 20 minutes
Walk/jog 4 miles in 48 minutes
Run 4 miles in 32 minutes
Swim 1800 yards in 48 minutes
Cycle 12 miles in 48 minutes

Other Benefits: Toward a Healthier Lifestyle

Executive Health Examiners has found that many executives who enter into a weight-control program based on exercise and diet are pleasantly surprised to find themselves changing their lifestyles in other ways. It seems to happen naturally. Time and again we have seen executives involved in exercise and weight-control programs cut down and then eliminate smoking, become more conscious about their eating habits, and cut back on excessive drinking. It all starts with the commitment to lose weight through an exercise-based program.

A 47-year-old investment banker provides a good example of this evolution toward a healthier lifestyle. When he came to Executive Health Examiners for a physical examination, he was 20 pounds overweight. He smoked a pack and a half of cigarettes a day, had a high cholesterol count and a high normal blood pressure reading of 140/90, and did not exercise regularly.

The banker's wife and teenage children all were involved in exercise programs, and he asked our doctors if jogging with his wife and kids would be good for him. His stress test was normal, and we advised him to begin his exercise program on his own but to start gradually.

The banker stopped smoking soon after he embarked on an aerobic walking-jogging exercise regimen. Family pressure helped him. His wife and kids threatened and cajoled until he finally gave in. Much to his surprise, he actually lost weight after giving up smoking. He thinks that his jogging program is the reason.

When the man came back to Executive Health Examiners

Many executives who enter into a weight-control program based on exercise and diet find themselves changing their lifestyles in other ways.

CALORIE AND EXERCISE EQUIVALENTS FOR POPULAR FOODS AND BEVERAGES

Food	Size/Serving	Approximate calories	Exercise required to burn it off[*]
Almonds	9–10 whole	70	2
Apple	$2\frac{1}{2}''$ diameter	70	2
Apple, baked with sugar	1 large	200	5
Applesauce, sweetened	$\frac{1}{2}$ cup	115	3
Apricots			
canned in water	$\frac{1}{2}$ cup	45	1
canned in syrup	$\frac{1}{2}$ cup	110	3
Apricots, dried	$\frac{1}{2}$ cup, 20 small halves	120	3
Asparagus	6 spears	20	1
Avocado	$\frac{1}{2}$ average	185	4
Bacon, fried	2 slices	90	2
Banana	1 average, $6'' = 1\frac{1}{2}''$	80	2
Beans, baked with pork in tomato sauce	$\frac{1}{2}$ cup	160	4
Beans (green, wax, or yellow)	$\frac{1}{2}$ cup	15	1
Beans, lima	$\frac{1}{2}$ cup	130	3
Beef			
corned, canned	3 oz.	185	4
hamburger, reg.	3 oz.	245	5
oven roast	3 oz., lean	200	5
pot roast	3 oz., lean	165	4
steak	3 oz., lean	175	4
Blueberries	$\frac{1}{2}$ cup, fresh	45	1
Bologna	2 oz., all meat	170	4
Bread			
white	1 slice 16 slices per loaf	75	2
whole-wheat	1 slice 16 slices per loaf	70	2
rye	1 slice 16 slices per loaf	70	2
Broccoli	$\frac{1}{2}$ cup	30	1
Butter	1 pat; 16 per $\frac{1}{4}$ pound	50	2
Cake			
chocolate with chocolate icing	2'' wedge of 10'' layer cake	345	8
plain cake without icing	$3'' \times 2'' \times 1\frac{1}{2}''$ slice	155	4
pound cake	$2\frac{3}{4}'' \times 3'' \times \frac{3}{8}''$	140	3
Candies			
caramels	3 medium	115	3
chocolate creams	2 or 3 small	110	3
fudge, milk chocolate	1 oz.	120	3
hard candy	1 oz.	110	3
milk chocolate	1-oz. bar	150	4
Cantaloupe	$\frac{1}{2}$ melon, 5'' diameter	60	2

[*] See the Exercise Selector on pages 159–160.

CALORIE AND EXERCISE EQUIVALENTS FOR POPULAR FOODS AND BEVERAGES (Continued)

Food	Size/Serving	Approximate calories	Exercise required to burn it off*
Carrot	5½" × 1" carrot	20	1
Celery	Two 8" stalks	10	1
Cereal			
corn flakes	1 cup	95	2
oatmeal	1 cup	130	3
wheat flakes	1 cup	105	3
Cheese			
American, processed	1 oz.	105	3
Cheddar, natural	1 oz.	115	3
cottage, creamed	1 oz.	30	1
Swiss	1 oz.	105	3
Cherries			
sweet, fresh	½ cup	40	1
sweet, canned with syrup	½ cup	105	3
Chicken	¼ small, broiled	185	4
Cookies	1 average	30	1
Corn	½ cup	70	2
Crab	½ cup, canned	85	2
Crackers			
graham	4 squares	55	2
rye wafers	2	45	1
saltines	Two 2" squares	35	1
Cucumber	¾" slice	5	1
Custard, baked	½ cup	140	3
Egg	1 large	80	2
Frankfurter	1 average	155	4
	1 with roll	245	5
Fruit cocktail	½ cup with syrup	100	3
Gelatin dessert	½ cup	70	2
Grapefruit	Half of 4¼" fruit	55	2
	½ cup canned with water	55	1
	½ cup canned with syrup	90	2
Gum, chewing	1 stick	10	1
Ham	3 oz., lean	160	4
Honeydew melon	½ fresh	50	2
Ice cream	½ cup	145	3
	soda, large	455	10
Ice milk	½ cup	110	3
Jam, jellies	1 tbsp.	55	2
Lamb	3 oz., lean	160	4
Lemonade	8-oz. glass	110	3
Lettuce	2 large leaves	10	1
Liver, beef	3 oz.	195	4
Macaroni	¾ cup, plain	115	3
	¾ cup, with cheese	360	8
Margarine	1 pat, 16 per ¼ pound	50	2

* See the Exercise Selector on pages 159–160.

CALORIE AND EXERCISE EQUIVALENTS FOR POPULAR FOODS AND BEVERAGES (Continued)

Food	Size/Serving	Approximate calories	Exercise required to burn it off*
Milk			
whole	1 cup	160	4
buttermilk	1 cup	90	2
half and half	1 tbsp.	20	1
skim	1 cup	90	2
chocolate	1 cup	210	5
chocolate milkshake	12 oz.	500	10
Muffin			
corn	2¾″ diameter	150	4
English	3½″ diameter	135	3
Noodles	¾ cup	150	4
Oil, salad	1 tbsp.	125	3
Orange juice	½ cup	55	2
Orange	3″ fruit	75	2
Pancake	4″ cake	55	2
Peach	2″ fruit, fresh	35	1
	½ cup, canned in syrup	100	3
Peanuts	2 tbsp.	105	3
Peanut butter	1 tbsp.	95	2
Pear	3″ × 2½″ fruit	100	3
Peas	½ cup	60	2
Pickle			
dill	1¾ × 4″	35	1
sweet	¾ × 1¾″	30	1
Pie			
fruit	⅛ of 9″ pie	300	7
lemon meringue	⅛ of 9″ pie	270	6
pecan	⅛ of 9″ pie	430	9
Pineapple	½ cup, fresh	40	1
	½ cup, canned	100	3
Plum	2″ fruit, fresh	25	1
	½ cup, canned	100	3
Popcorn	1 cup	40	1
Pork	3 oz., lean	230	5
Potato chips	10 medium	115	3
Potato			
baked	2½, 5 oz.	90	2
french fried	Ten 2″-long pieces	155	4
mashed	½ cup	90	2
sweet	5″ × 2″, 6 oz.	155	4
Pretzels	5 small sticks	20	1
Prunes	1½ cup, unsweetened	150	4
Radishes	4 small	5	1
Raisins	½ cup	230	5
Rice, cooked	¾ cup	140	3

* See the Exercise Selector on pages 159–160.

CALORIE AND EXERCISE EQUIVALENTS FOR POPULAR FOODS AND BEVERAGES
(Continued)

Food	Size/Serving	Approximate calories	Exercise required to burn it off*
Salad dressing			
blue cheese	1 tbsp.	75	2
French	1 tbsp.	65	2
low-calorie	1 tbsp.	15	1
mayonnaise	1 tbsp.	100	3
Thousand Island	1 tbsp.	125	3
Salmon	3 oz., canned	120	3
Sausage, pork	2 oz.	270	6
Sherbet	½ cup	130	3
Shrimp	3 oz., 17 medium canned	100	3
Soft drink			
cola	12-oz. can	145	3
fruit flavors	12-oz. can	170	4
ginger ale	12-oz. can	115	3
root beer	12-oz. can	150	4
Soup			
bouillon	1 cup	30	1
chicken noodle	1 cup	60	2
cream of mushroom	1 cup	155	3
minestrone	1 cup	105	3
tomato	1 cup, made with water	90	2
	1 cup, made with milk	180	4
Spaghetti			
plain	¾ cup	115	3
with tomato sauce	¾ cup	195	4
with meatballs	¾ cup	250	6
Spinach	½ cup	20	1
Strawberries	½ cup, fresh	30	1
	½ cup, frozen	140	3
Sugar	1 tsp.	15	1
Tomato juice	½ cup	20	1
Tuna	3 oz., canned	170	4
Turkey	3 oz., light meat	150	4
	3 oz., dark meat	175	4
Veal	3 oz., lean	185	4
Waffle	1 average	210	5
Watermelon	one 2-lb. wedge	115	3
Yogurt	1 cup, plain	120	3
	1 cup, with fruit	260	6

* See the Exercise Selector on pages 159–160.

12 months later for a physical exam, we found that he had lost 21 pounds, that his cholesterol level was down, and that his blood pressure had dropped to 135/85. He said he felt better about himself psychologically. He also felt more productive professionally and reported that his jogging had enhanced his family life. He was spending more time with his family on the running track where they all worked out. He looked better, felt better about himself, and felt he had more energy during the day. Best of all, he was able to eliminate smoking. It's easy to see that all these improvements were sparked by the man's decision to lose weight through diet and exercise.

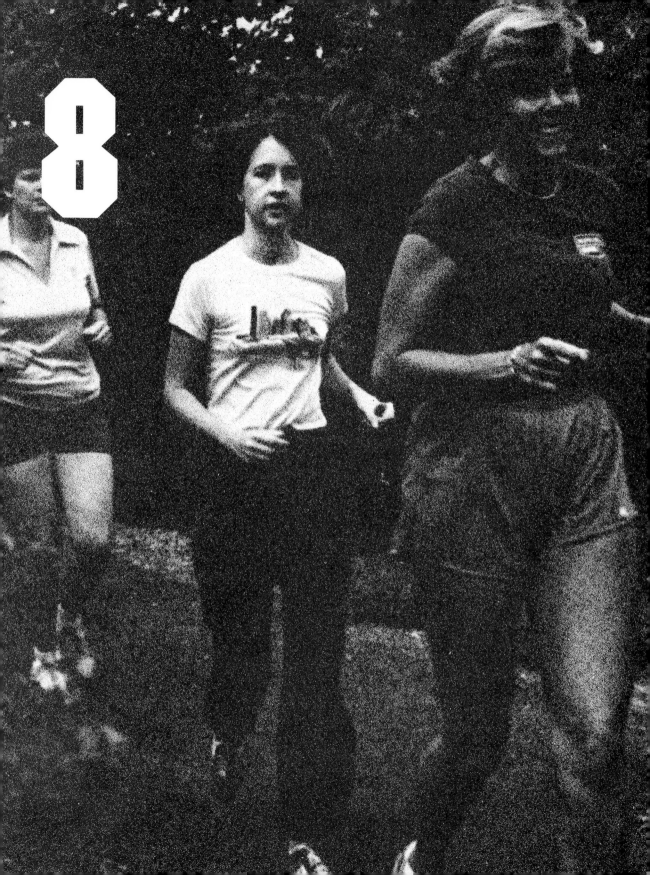

8

EXERCISE AND THE WOMAN EXECUTIVE

A 46-year-old vice president of an investment firm recently asked EHE doctors whether she needed to go on an exercise program. "I've heard that women are far less likely to have heart attacks than men," she said. "And I'm in fairly decent shape. Do I really need to spend time exercising?" The answer our doctors gave was, of course, a resounding yes. The pressures and demands of the executive lifestyle do not discriminate by sex. Woman executives suffer from the same job-related mental and physical ailments that plague their male counterparts. Both men and women executives need to build their cardiovascular and musculoskeletal systems through a carefully prescribed balanced exercise regimen.

There are significant physiological differences between men and women, but there is no essential difference in terms of the cardiovascular system, respiratory capacity, or metabolism. Women have the same capability as men of developing athletic skills such as dexterity, agility, coordination, and cardiovascular training. But only in recent years, following the nationwide exercise boom, have large num-

The pressures and demands of the executive lifestyle do not discriminate by sex.

THE BENEFITS OF EXERCISING FOR WOMEN

The beneficial effects of regular physical exercise on the heart, lungs, bones and muscles are well known. Less publicized benefits are an improved sense of well-being, weight loss, weight control, and decreased menstrual pain and discomfort. . . . These combined advantages of regular exercise far outweigh any potential reproductive hazards.

Mona Shangold, M.D.

bers of women begun to participate in exercise and sports. Margaret Dunkle, a leading expert on women in athletics, explained part of the reason: "Women have not been encouraged to participate in athletics at least partly because the traits associated with athletic excellence—achievement, self-confidence, aggressiveness, leadership strength, swiftness—are often seen as being in 'contradiction' with the role of women."[1] These traits once were reserved only for men, but today they fit the profile of most successful executives, male or female.

Physiological Differences

Of course there are significant differences between men and women, but none of the unique feminine characteristics prevents women from taking part in, and benefiting from, exercise. The most important physiological factor determining human athletic ability is the effect of hormones on the physical maturation process. All male and female bodies contain estrogen, the female hormone, and testosterone, the male hormone. Men have a much higher ratio of testosterone; women, a significantly greater amount of estrogen. Boys and girls mature nearly evenly until about age 10. Then, during the next 5 to 6 years, girls

Women have not been encouraged to participate in athletics at least partly because the traits associated with athletic excellence are often seen as being in contradiction with the role of women.

[1] Margaret Dunkle, "What Constitutes Equality For Women in Sports," Washington, D.C., Project on the Status and Education of Women, September 1975, p. 21.

None of the unique characteristics of men and women should prevent them from exercising.

undergo rapid physical maturation. During this time boys also are maturing, but not as rapidly as girls.

Men reach their maximum growth at around age 20. The longer, slower growth in men results primarily in more defined muscles, especially in the upper body and arms; it also is responsible for masculine secondary sex characteristics, including a lower voice and facial hair. The rapid female maturation process causes most women to have lower centers of gravity than men, because more weight is concentrated in women's thighs and hips. Thus, the only innate physical advantage men have over women is a stronger upper body.

The upper bodies of men have larger bone and greater articular surfaces than the upper bodies of women. This gives men a mechanical and structural advantage over women in sports such as football and baseball, which require upper body strength, but there is no advantage for men over women in aerobic or flexibility exercises. Men's "longer bones act as greater lever arms, producing more force for sports requiring striking, hitting or kicking," writes Dr. Letha Yurko Hunter, assistant professor of orthopedics at the University of Washington.[2] Men also have more muscle mass than women: about 40 percent of total body weight compared to about 23 percent. Women have a heavier proportion of body fat: from 22 to 25 percent of body weight, compared with men, who have 14 percent. Women also have slightly lower metabolic rates than men.

The most obvious differences between men and women are seen in the reproductive systems. These differences have given rise to a number of myths involving women and exercise, all of which have been proved untrue.

[2] Letha Yurko Hunter, "The Female Athlete," *Medical Times*, June 1981.

Reproductive Organs and Breasts One widely held myth is that taking part in exercise is harmful to a woman's reproductive organs and breasts. Doctors say that there is virtually no risk of harming the female sexual organs during physical activity. As Dorothy Harris, director of the Center for Women and Sport at Pennsylvania State University, says, a woman has "more natural protection for contact sports than a man; she has a subcutaneous layer of fat protecting the muscles and joints and her sex organs are internal, making them practically invulnerable to injury."

Although some women report sore or tender breasts after exercising, much of that discomfort can be relieved by wearing a specially designed sports bra. Many types are now on the market. Exercise does not contribute to sagging breasts, by the way. Many forms of exercise, especially those involving the arms, can strengthen the pectoral muscles, thus improving posture and breast contour.

Postchildbirth Some people believe that a woman's athletic abilities decline after childbirth, but again, there is no scientific evidence to prove the allegation. "There is no

Executive Health Examiners has found that pregnant women can exercise safely for nearly the entire term of pregnancy.

> # World records have been set and Olympic gold medals won by women during all stages of the menstrual cycle.

need to restrict physical activity for women in any manner whatsoever," says athletic trainer Joan Gillette. "There . . . are no ill effects during pregnancy, delivery or later on. . . . Women athletes receive injuries due to the lack of proper conditioning and poor coaching."

Menstruation Another myth holds that a woman cannot exert maximum physical strength during menstruation. However, world records have been set and Olympic gold medals won by women during all stages of the menstrual cycle, and mild menstruation should not prevent a woman from doing her everyday exercise routine.

Amenorrhea, which is a medical term for the absence of menstrual periods, and other menstrual irregularities are often blamed on exercise, but that myth has been dispelled by Mona Shangold, M.D., professor of obstetrics and gynecology at the Albert Einstein College of Medicine in New York. Dr. Shangold, an expert on the effects of exercise on the female reproductive system, wrote recently: "Despite alarming claims of menstrual irregularity in athletes, it has not been proved that exercise is responsible or harmful. For women who do experience irregular menstrual periods when they exercise heavily, it should never be assumed that the problem is exercise related—or that it is not serious." Dr. Shangold recommends that women experiencing amenorrhea or other menstrual abnormalities consult their gynecologists.

Executive Health Examiners has found that women involved in EHE-recommended exercise programs report that exercise decreases premenstrual tension and physical symptoms such as cramps and bloating. "The months

The bottom line on the subject of exercising and menstruation is to use common sense.

when I do active physical exercise, I experience no menstrual discomfort whatsoever," said a 32-year-old advertising executive. "When I don't do any exercising, I'm in agony. I get cramps, bloating, and it's just misery. It's the best motivation I can think of to do my exercises regularly."

The bottom line on the subject of exercising and menstruation is to use common sense. If your period is particularly heavy, do not exercise; the same is true if you have a heavy cold or a sprained ankle. But remember that most women can exercise normally during normal menstruation. As Dr. Shangold sums it up:

> The beneficial effects of regular physical exercise on the heart, lungs, bones and muscles are well-known. Less publicized benefits are an improved sense of well-being, weight loss, weight control, and decreased menstrual pain and discomfort. . . . These combined advantages of regular exercises far outweigh any potential reproductive hazards.

Pregnancy

Executive Health Examiners has found that pregnant women can exercise safely for nearly the entire term of pregnancy, but we strongly recommend that pregnant women consult a physician about the types of exercise they undertake. Again, common sense dictates that women should moderate their exercise regimens during the late stages of pregnancy.

According to a survey conducted by Dr. David A. Leaf of Portland, Oregon, pregnant women respond to exercise in much the same way as women who are not pregnant.

There is even some evidence, Dr. Leaf reported to a Northwest Sports Medicine and Conditioning Seminar, that exercising mothers may have shorter periods of labor than mothers who do not exercise. No evidence has been found that running or other aerobic exercises harm the developing fetus. Nevertheless, it is very important that pregnant women avoid excessive fatigue and consult a doctor about their exercise routines during the entire term.

The Muscle Controversy

Perhaps the biggest myth that has kept women from exercising is the fear that they will develop large, "unfeminine" muscles, although it has been proved medically that women can greatly increase their strength through weight lifting without building large, bulky muscles. The reason is that most women do not produce male hormones in sufficient quantity to develop large muscles.

The leading expert in this field is Dr. Jack Wilmore of the Department of Physical Education at the University of Arizona. His experiments in this area involved 10-week weight-training programs with groups of untrained college-age men and women. Dr. Wilmore found that while men are able to lift heavier weights than women, the male/female ratios all but disappear when considered in relation to overall body weight. We've always been told that women are so much weaker than men, but Dr. Wilmore's experiments show that they have almost exactly the same strength.

Wilmore's experiments also showed that women's

Women can practice weight lifting without building large, bulky muscles.

muscles, while increasing in strength, did not significantly increase in size. The studies showed that women generally developed one-tenth the muscle size of men who worked out in the same weight program. Women's biceps grew an average of only about one-fourth of an inch, while their strength improved 11 to 30 percent.

The results of a study of men and women volunteers at Oregon State University who used a special technique of weight training called power lifting correlated with Dr. Wilmore's findings. Women and men have "the same physiological ability . . . to tolerate and adapt to" the demands of power lifting, according to Oregon State professor of physical education John P. O'Shea and his assistant Julie Wegner, who oversaw the study. O'Shea and Wegner found that there is no medical or scientific basis for the myth that women "lack the physical capacity to respond to strength training." They concluded that while "it is true that women have less muscle mass than men per unit of body weight and bone density and consequently do not possess the same absolute strength potential as men, women can develop strength relative to their own physical potential."[3]

Women, Stress, and Exercise

Women executives are subject to the same stresses on the job that men face, and many women executives have the additional pressure of balancing home, family, and work. "A woman who feels that she must take primary responsibility for her marriage and family as well as manage a career—a Superwoman—is setting herself up for failure in one or another of these spheres," said Ruth Weeks, M.D., a psychiatrist at the University of Virginia Medical Center. "Disappointment, lowered self-esteem and depression are going to be the result."[4]

There is no conclusive evidence that women executives are more prone than men to cardiopulmonary dis-

[3] John P. O'Shea and Julie Wegner, "Power Weight Training and the Female Athlete," *The Physician and Sportsmedicine*, June 1981, p. 120.
[4] *Working Woman*, January 1980, p. 51.

eases. A 1980 survey conducted by the Heart, Lung and Blood Institute of the National Institutes of Health found that professional women are less likely to develop heart disease than women clerical workers and that women as a group have lower rates of coronary heart disease than men.

But a Stanford University study released in January 1981 found that young women executives with master's degrees in business "showed significantly more psychological and physical signs of stress" than their male counterparts. Four times as many of the women sought psychological counseling. As Chicago psychiatrist Irvin H. Gracer put it, "If women executives attempt to emulate the emotional patterns of their male peers and restrain their tendencies to be open and candid about how they feel, they also may pay the penalty that men pay."[5] Dr. Gracer left out one other option for women executives facing stress on the job. They can begin balanced exercise programs that can go a long way toward ameliorating the effects of stress on any executive, male or female.

[5] Quoted in Jane Adams, *Woman on Top* (New York: Hawthorn Books, 1979), p. 173.

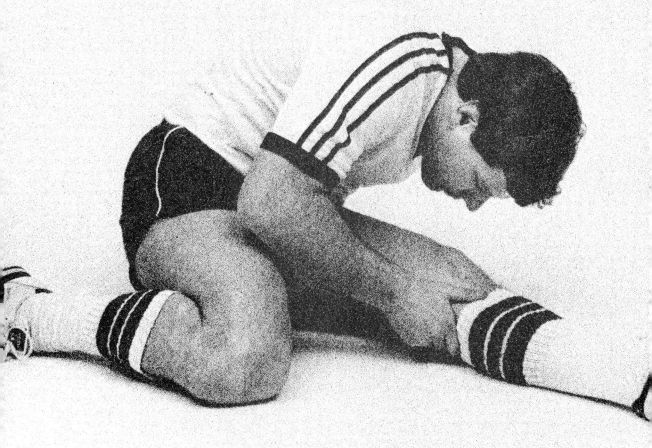

HOW TO AVOID INJURY

Injuries and exercise go together. The odds are that if you embark on an exercise program involving aerobics, stretching, and strength building, sooner or later you will suffer some sort of injury. The most common injuries are relatively minor, and there are commonsense steps you can take to greatly minimize your chances of developing serious injuries. If you feel a twinge in your knee while running, slow down. If the pain persists, slow to a walk and give your leg a rest. Most injuries are caused by overuse, by doing too much exercise with too much intensity in too short a period of time. The way to avoid the consequences of overuse injuries is to use your head. Warm up slowly and gradually for at least 10 minutes before aerobic exercises, decrease the intensity at the first sign of trouble, and stop completely if pain persists.

Another way to minimize the risk of injury is to choose equipment designed to come between your body and injuries. The most important piece of equipment in running and walking is the shoe.

The most common sports injuries are relatively minor.

Running and Walking Shoes: What to Look For

One of the prime benefits of the physical fitness explosion of the mid-1970s for American joggers and walkers has been the parallel expansion and availability of scientifically designed exercise shoes. There are at least twenty brands of excellent athletic shoes on the market today, ranging in price from under $20 to over $75, and there are many different types of special athletic shoes from which to choose. There are running shoes that are perfectly suitable for walking. There are basketball shoes, baseball shoes, track shoes, tennis shoes, golf shoes, and so on.

One question frequently asked EHE doctors by executives about to embark on jogging programs involves what type of shoe to buy. "*Running Times* magazine gives out 'gold shoe' awards to some brands that don't even make *Runner's World* magazine's 'highly recommended' list," an advertising executive complained to our doctors recently. "How am I supposed to know what brand and model to buy?"

The answer to that question is that even though buying running shoes is an individual decision, there are several things everyone should consider before selecting a pair. First, buy a shoe especially made for running; basketball or tennis shoes will not do. Any of the major brands such as Adidas, Nike, Puma, New Balance, Converse, Tiger, Patrik, and Etonic are acceptable. Executive Health Examiners recommends buying running shoes from a store that specializes in athletic footwear.

Talk to the salesperson and discuss exactly what you will be using the shoes for. Especially important is the kind of surface you will be running on and how many miles a week you will be running. Try on several pair of shoes, because the most important criterion is how they feel on you. Remember to wear the same type of socks you will be running in. One important thing to check is how the heel fits; it should be stable and fit snugly, but not too tightly. If you are used to wearing a built-up heel, buy a pair of running shoes with that feature. If your street shoes are flat, go with running shoes with low heels. You should also make sure there is room between your toes and the tips of the shoes. The shoes also should be flexible and have well-padded soles.

Footwear for Cycling, Stretching, and Weight Lifting

Choosing the type of footwear for the other exercises in your routine is not as crucial as it is for running and walking, because your feet and legs take the most pounding in running and walking. (If you choose rope skipping, use running shoes.) For both indoor and outdoor cycling, all you need is a good pair of basketball or tennis sneakers. Do not use running shoes on rolling bicycles, because the waffle soles can get caught in the pedals, and do not wear sandals or high heels.

Bicycle specialty stores sell shoes designed to be worn while cycling, but these shoes are designed for serious race cyclists and are by no means necessary for the cyclist interested only in exercise. The same holds true for stretching and strength-building exercises. You can buy special gym shoes for these exercises, but it's perfectly all right to wear sneakers. If you are doing your stretching and strength building in the same sessions as your aerobics, you can either warm up and cool down indoors without shoes or use the same shoes you use for aerobic exercises if you work out outdoors.

Clothing

The next time you are out on the jogging path or bike path, look around. You will notice that the basic running and cycling outfits consist of T-shirts and shorts in the spring and summer and sweat suits or warmup suits in fall and winter. That is about all you have to know in the area of exercise clothing.

Executive Health Examiners recommends that you wear loose and comfortable clothing made of natural fibers to facilitate comfort. Cotton or wool shirts, shorts, and pants "breathe," whereas synthetic fabrics hold in perspiration.

You will therefore be much more comfortable in cotton or wool. Nylon running shorts are best for hot weather because they are extremely lightweight.

The layered look is still fashionable for exercise in cold weather. Try a T-shirt covered by a sweat shirt or warmup jacket, but it's not necessary to worry about protecting yourself from cold weather until the temperature dips below freezing. Once you start running, walking, or cycling, your body will adapt well to temperature in the 40s and 50s; in fact, long-distance runners say that 55 degrees is about the perfect temperature for running. When the thermometer dips below freezing, you should protect your hands and head. We recommend lightweight wool or cotton gloves and caps.

Clothing for Cyclists

There are many different types of clothes made especially for cyclists. You can buy a special head-to-foot cycling outfit complete with shoes, socks, pants, shirt, cap, and gloves, but the average exercise cyclist can wear any comfortable clothing so long as the outfit does not restrict movement. The black cotton skin-tight cycling shorts that racers wear have a special inner lining designed to cushion road bumps, but most of those who cycle for exercise do not need these shorts. If you find yourself logging lots of miles on your bike, you might think about getting a pair. Shorts and a T-shirt are *de rigueur* for warm weather; the layered look, for cool weather. In the winter, it's best to wear a pair of gloves, because your hands bear the brunt of the cold.

There is some mandatory equipment for outdoor cyclists. A helmet is a smart investment. More than one experienced cyclist has wound up in the hospital, and some have been killed, from falling off a ten-speed bike. Something as seemingly innocuous as a wet leaf can cause a fall. If your head is not protected, you are asking for trouble. There are many types of helmets to choose from. The best ones are lightweight and have tinted adjustable visors.

There is some other equipment rolling bicyclists should not be without: a lightweight backpack or saddlepack to carry extra clothing, rain gear for an emergency, some sort of clip to keep your pants legs out of the chains, a tool bag and pump to handle road repairs, a headlight, and front, rear, and wheel reflectors to make yourself visible at night.

Clothing for Swimming, Rope Skipping, and Yoga

Swimming, of course, requires only a good swimsuit that clings to your body but does not cut off circulation. For rope skipping, lose-fitting but not bellowing clothing will do. Again, you cannot go wrong with shorts and a T-shirt. The same is true for strength-building exercises. For stretching, and especially for yoga, loose and comfortable clothing is the rule; women can wear leotards.

Avoiding Injuries

There is an entire branch of medicine devoted to sports. The science of sports medicine has grown markedly in the last decade, and those of us who exercise are among the beneficiaries of the gains in knowledge about injuries and injury prevention. We now know that most injuries are caused by overuse. Thus it is vital that you warm up before beginning your aerobic, strength-building, and stretching exercises. It is equally vital to cool down afterward. It also is important to increase your times and distances gradually.

If you do not use these commonsense procedures, chances are, you will suffer an injury similar to the one that befell an EHE patient who increased his running time too quickly after beginning his program. This man, a physician

The science of sports medicine has grown markedly in the last decade.

in his late forties, noticed great improvement in his cardio-vascular capacity after 4 weeks of running regularly. He began increasing his distances nearly every time he ran, but within a month he complained to EHE doctors that he had severe pain in his knees and that his hamstring muscles were constantly sore. When we found out how long he ran every day, we immediately advised him to refrain from running entirely for a month. After the 4-week enforced rest, we set him up on a new running program designed for gradual progress. He began to warm up slowly and gradually and stayed on the timetable. His leg problems soon disappeared.

The Most Common Sports Injuries

As you might assume, leg and foot problems are the most common injuries associated with exercise. According to a study done by a Lenox Hill Hospital clinic that treats primarily recreational athletes in New York City, the most frequent injuries involve knees, ankles, and shoulders. Knee injuries, in fact, accounted for nearly half of all problems.

Other studies of exercise-related injuries similarly indicate that the knee is one of the most vulnerable parts of the body, an extremely fragile joint commonly injuried in many sports, including cycling. Extensive uphill pedaling puts tremendous pressure on the middle surface of the kneecap. This can cause what is also the most common runner's injury: inflammation of the cartilage behind the kneecap, commonly known as runner's knee. The knee "is simply not designed for most of the things people want to do with it today," says Robert Kerlan, M.D., director of the National Athletic Health Institute in Inglewood, California, and an expert on knee injuries.

Leg and foot problems are the most common injuries associated with exercise.

AN INJURY SURVEY AT LENOX HILL HOSPITAL, 1975 TO 1979

Injuries to Urban Recreational Athletes			Sports in which Injuries Occurred		
Body Part	*No.*	*%*	*Sport*	*No.*	*%*
Knee	486	45.5	Running/ jogging	340	32.6
Ankle	105	9.8	Basketball	101	9.7
Shoulder	82	7.7	Tennis	97	9.3
Foot/heel	77	7.2	Ballet/dancing	74	7.1
Elbow	63	5.9	Football	44	4.2
Back	53	5.0	Snow skiing	37	3.5
Hip	48	4.5	Weight lifting	36	3.4
Tibia	47	4.4	Baseball/ softball	32	3.1
Femur/ hamstring	44	4.1	Martial arts	31	3.0
Fibula/calf	19	1.8	Soccer	16	1.5
Wrist	17	1.6	Gymnastics	14	1.3
Neck	9	0.8	Ice hockey	11	1.1
Pelvis	7	0.7	Miscellaneous (35 sports)	133	12.7
Groin	4	0.4	Unspecified	78	7.5
Finger	2	0.2			
Humerus	2	0.2			
Leg (unspecified)	2	0.2	**Total**	1,044*	100.0
Total	1,067	100.0			

* Some athletes did not identify any sport and some identified more than one.

Philip A. Witman, et al., "Common Problems Seen in a Metropolitan Sports Injury Clinic," *The Physician and Sportsmedicine*, March 1981, p. 106.

Preventing Injuries

Doing special strength-building exercises, running on smooth surfaces, warming up the leg muscles well, and choosing good running shoes are the best ways to avoid not only knee but other common leg problems associated with exercise. These include stress fractures, bone bruises, shin splints (the aching of inflamed muscles or tendons in the lower legs), inflammation of the Achilles tendon, and bone spurs of the heel.

Another preventive measure involves a fairly new type of sports medicine called orthotics. A group of podiatrists now specializes in fitting runners, cyclists, and walkers with orthotic devices, which are molds designed from your foot to fit into your running shoes. The object is to balance the foot in a neutral position while you exercise. These lightweight devices are made of plastic, rubber, or leather and can be custom-made to correct many of the various leg problems. Orthotic devices, which cost as much as $150, are not recommended for everyone, but if you have recurring leg problems, consult a podiatrist or othopedist and ask whether such a device will provide you with relief.

To repeat, for leg problems, the most important things you can do to lessen the risk of serious injury are to:

* *Buy a well-built, comfortable pair of running shoes*

* *Run or walk on a smooth and, if possible, pliable surface*

* *Warm up slowly, progress gradually, and cool down slowly*

* *See a podiatrist or orthopedist for an orthotic device if you have continuing problems*

There are other problems associated with running that have nothing to do with the legs but that for the most part are avoidable with some commonsense preventive techniques. Doctors have uncovered what is believed to be a benign condition in many joggers: athletic pseudonephritis, or "jogger's kidney." The symptoms are abnormal levels of protein, red blood cells, and other substances in the urine. The condition may be caused by reduction of blood flow to the kidneys during an hour or more of jogging. The condition cures itself within 2 days, but doctors do not know whether it leads to kidney damage. If you think you are suffering from this condition, it's best to consult a physician and cut back on your running time.

"Runner's nipple" is caused when clothing rubs against the sensitive areas of the breasts. This condition can affect men and women, and although it is not a serious problem, runner's nipple can be very painful. It primarily affects long-distance runners. The remedy: applying ointment to the breasts before running or taping on gauze pads for protection. A good running bra takes care of the problem for women.

Careful, well thought out exercise programs can minimize most of the dangers of injury.

In summary, there is an ever-present risk of injury when you are exercising, but there are ways to minimize the risk. Careful, well thought out exercise programs can minimize most of the potential dangers, and Executive Health Examiners believes that the potential benefits of regular exercise—especially for those who live largely sedentary lives—far outweigh the risks of physical injury.

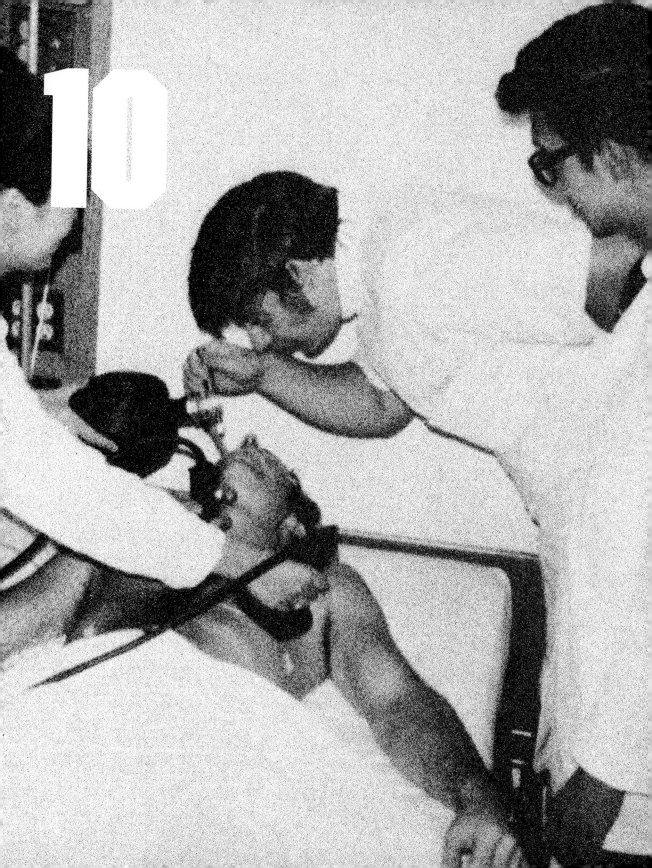

HEART DISEASE, DIABETES, AND ASTHMA: THE VALUE OF EXERCISE

Is it possible for executives with heart disease to undertake an exercise program safely? The answer is a qualified yes. It is possible for recovering heart attack patients to undertake such a program, but not without clearance from their personal physicians and cardiologists.

More and more doctors are finding that exercise can be beneficial to a recovering heart patient. A real estate executive had a massive heart attack not long after he retired 3 years ago at age 69. He came through a double-bypass operation and 3 months later was fitted with a pacemaker. Three

---

More doctors are finding that exercise can be beneficial to a recovering heart attack patient.

---

months after that he enrolled in a cardiac rehabilitation program that emphasized daily walking and thrice-weekly workouts on a stationary bicycle.

His exercise sessions were directed by a trained nurse who monitored her exercising patients' heartbeat and other vital signs. Progress reports were sent to the patients' cardiologists. "I can't say enough about my exercise program," the executive said recently. "It makes me feel stronger and healthier. Our nurse works very closely with the doctors, and any time there is the slightest problem, my cardiologist calls me in for an examination."

After 2 months of cardiac rehabilitation, this man felt well enough to return to his normal daily activities. This case is not atypical. Younger recovering heart attack patients often return to work in a matter of weeks after beginning cardiac rehabilitation programs, and they return in good physical and mental condition. "It is my belief that, with a professionally supervised exercise program, many heart attack victims may not just return to work, but they may restore their hearts to a state far better than before the heart attack, and so prevent subsequent attacks," writes Robert C. Cantu, M.D., of the Emerson Hospital in Concord, Massachusetts.[1] Dr. Cantu and other experts are quick to point out, however, that cardiac rehabilitation is not complete unless obvious cardiac risk factors—hypertension, obesity, cigarette smoking, including the sedentary lifestyle—are eliminated or tightly controlled.

Exercise After a Heart Attack

Terence Kavanaugh, M.D., of the Toronto Rehabilitation Center, has specialized in treating post-heart attack patients with exercise therapy. His program takes patients as early as 6 weeks after their heart attacks and concentrates on walking and running. A group of Dr. Kavanaugh's patients made history in 1973 when they entered and completed the Boston Marathon. The seven middle-aged former heart attack victims who ran in the marathon were monitored by Dr. Ka-

---

[1] Robert C. Cantu, *Toward Fitness* (Human Sciences Press, 1980), pp. 135–136.

vanaugh throughout the race. They reported no respiratory problems.

Jack Scaff, M.D., of Honolulu also specializes in exercise programs for postcardiac patients. Since 1973 he has entered more than 1000 of his patients in the Honolulu Marathon. As is the case with Dr. Kavanaugh's charges, Dr. Scaff's runners are constantly monitored and train especially for the marathon for many months. None of his runners has had any serious cardiac complications.

"These feats are important as dramatic illustrations of the value of the medically supervised post-heart attack exercise program," Dr. Cantu writes. "They point out just how far one's exercise prescription can be upgraded if one desires to put in the time and effort. But it is certainly not necessary to make such a commitment. A program just three or four hours a week is sufficient to gain the physiological and psychological benefits desired."

Exercise programs for postcardiac patients should be taken under the close supervision of cardiologists. Especially important is the time to begin initial exercising. In the past, the accepted medical thinking was to give cardiac patients as much bed rest as possible. They were told to avoid straining and were cautioned to avoid such comparatively easy tasks as climbing stairs.

In the last decade medical thinking has changed on the subject of when heart attack patients should begin exercising. Many doctors now advise beginning an exercise program as soon as the patient has recovered enough strength to handle light walking. Although Dr. Kavanaugh's Toronto program takes patients as early as 6 weeks after their heart attacks, some doctors encourage patients to begin exercise programs even earlier.

Many doctors advise beginning an exercise program as soon as the cardiac patient has recovered enough strength for light walking.

A 1981 study of staff members of the University of Washington's Division of Cardiology examined the effects of early exercise programs on patients who had acute myocardial infarction. The conclusion was that while such low-intensity exercise programs do not improve the health of patients, they also do not have any demonstrable deleterious effects. The conclusion was optimistic: "If one assumes that a sedentary lifestyle is a risk factor and that exercise is a desirable preventive measure, then starting an exercise program during hospitalization when patients are highly motivated may well help to establish a habit of exercise."[2]

Other Diseases and Exercise

Many executives are concerned about physical problems other than injuries or heart attacks when embarking on an exercise program. "Doctor, I have diabetes. Does this mean I can't exercise on a regular basis?" This is a question EHE doctors often hear. There is one rule of thumb concerning exercise and diseases such as diabetes, asthma, and arthritis: The patient must be ultraconscious of his or her particular disease while exercising. If there is the slightest sign of any abnormality, we strongly recommend that you immediately consult your physician. From our experience with setting up exercise programs for hundreds of executives with various diseases, here are some specific recommendations.

Diabetes Executive Health Examiners has found that exercise can benefit most diabetic patients. We have treated diabetic patients who, after adopting a regular exercise program, have been able to decrease their insulin requirements. There are even cases of people with adult-onset diabetes who no longer needed insulin after adopting an exercise regimen.

"Quite clearly, the vast majority of epidemiological and clinical studies lend credence to the belief that regular physical activity promotes good health and these observations are supported by the physiologic changes which can be

[2] Erika S. Sivarajan, et al., *New England Journal of Medicine*, August 13, 1981.

> # After adopting a regular exercise program, diabetic patients have been able to decrease their insulin requirements.

documented in an actively exercising individual," writes Dr. Thomas M. Flood of the Joslin Diabetes Foundation in Boston. Dr. Flood warns, however, that any diabetic about to embark on an exercise program should work closely with his or her physician to set up a regimen tailored to the patient's particular condition. "Observation of a few common sense rules," Dr. Flood writes, "with special attention to diet and potential insulin changes during the early, evolutionary stages of an exercise program, will . . . enable diabetic patients to derive greater benefit from their exercise."[3]

Arthritis We do not recommend running for arthritic patients with hip or knee conditions. Swimming is ideal for those problems. The best choice for the arthritic patient is a program in which the affected joints are not exposed to potential damage. People suffering from rheumatoid arthritis should not begin an exercise program without consulting a physical rehabilitation specialist.

It now appears that contrary to popular opinion, runners, cyclists, and other regular exercisers do not have greater risk of developing osteoarthritis. However, there is some evidence that specific joint injuries can cause this form of arthritis, and so it is especially important to have severe joint injuries attended to quickly and thoroughly.

Asthma There is no reason why a person with asthma cannot take part in a balanced exercise program. One word of warning, though. Exercising in extremely cold or polluted air can trigger an asthma attack. It is very important for those with asthma to warm up thoroughly before exercising and to begin aerobic exercises slowly and gradually.

[3] Thomas M. Flood, *Medical Times*, May 1980, p. 85.

There is no reason why a person with asthma cannot take part in a balanced exercise program.

Doctors at the University of Western Australia in Nedlands have found that exercise, when undertaken with a physician's permission and with commonsense precautions, can help most asthmatics. Research shows that:

> Even persons with moderately severe asthma can often participate [in exercise] if a few simple guidelines are followed. Regular vigorous activity has been shown to bring several benefits, including increased physical fitness, enhanced tolerance of attacks and a greater social and psychological independence. Far from being a barrier to involvement in physical pursuits, asthma should perhaps indicate an even greater need for such involvement.[4]

Lower Back Pain Most lower back pain is preventable, and the secret is usually exercise. For some back pain, including herniated disks, no exercise should be done without consulting a physician, but for most lower back problems stretching exercises often provide relief. "From a preventive standpoint [exercise] is one of the simplest and most important prescriptions for a healthy back," EHE director Dr. Richard E. Winter has written. "Low back pain for millions of Americans is simply another health concern for which we have responsibility and, fortunately, over which we can exercise control."[5]

There are a number of specific exercise programs offered at places like YMCAs that are designed to focus on strengthening back muscles and alleviating back pain. Yoga exercises concentrate on the back muscles, but it is important to remember to consult your exercise instructor or yoga teacher before undertaking a program.

[4] Alan R. Morton, et al., *The Physician and Sportsmedicine*, March 1981, p. 59.
[5] Richard E. Winter, *Over 40*, November 1978, p. 50.

Hypertension High blood pressure is one of the risk factors associated with cardiovascular disease. In cases of mild to moderate hypertension, a regular aerobic exercise program can be a valuable supplement to the treatment routine. Approval from your physician is necessary before starting such a program. Since exercise programs usually reduce weight and combat stress, they also can lead to lowered blood pressure. EHE medical records contain evidence of many patients who experienced a lowering of blood pressure after 6 to 12 months of exercising. There is no direct proof that the exercise leads directly to the lowered blood pressure, but we believe there is a correlation.

It's a Lifetime Commitment

It's customary in books of this kind to conclude with an exhortation designed to encourage the reader to begin an exercise program immediately. Before we get to that, we would like to present a few sobering thoughts.

First of all, exercise is a lifetime commitment. It's not a fad or something to dabble in when the mood strikes. In order to get the full benefits of exercise, you need to practice all three components on a regular basis. If you stop, you will lose nearly everything you have gained. This is especially true for aerobics exercises, but it also goes for the stretching and strength-building components of the exercise program.

Executive Health Examiners has found that the number one reason executives abandon exercise programs is boredom. "I just can't stand to pedal that damn stationary bike one more minute," an exasperated New Jersey insurance ex-

The number one reason why executives abandon exercise programs is boredom.

ecutive told EHE doctors recently. "I've been pedaling diligently three times a week for a year and a half, and I can't take staring at the walls any longer."

Combating Boredom

The answer for this woman and for all others who become bored with their regular exercise routines is to find ways to make exercise sessions enjoyable. If your exercise is fun, you will look forward to doing it. For bored indoor cyclists, we suggest moving the bike in front of the TV or radio or buying a portable tape recorder so that you can listen to music while pedaling.

Another way to combat boredom is to vary your routines slightly without abandoning them altogether. Runners, walkers, and outdoor cyclists can change their routes or the time of day they venture forth. You can vary your aerobic routines according to the season, switching to running in warmer weather and indoor cycling during cold weather, for example.

You can exercise with friends to alleviate boredom. Since the pace of aerobic exercises is designed so that you can hold a normal conversation, running, walking, and cycling are perfect for two people to exercise and chat at the same time. Any time you have company during your usually solitary exercise routine, a bit of adrenaline pumps into your system and you seem to glide effortlessly through the routine. This is good so long as you do not overdo it and go beyond your capacity.

We have suggested getting family members involved in exercise routines. Cajoling a lazy spouse out of bed at 6 A.M. will not only get you an exercise partner but will also give you a chance to show your partner what you are doing in the early hours of the morning.

Most exercisers find that after several months they begin changing their routines naturally. They find themselves adding twists, abandoning others, inventing new types of stretches, running in unexplored directions, and exercising at different times of the day. Some executives have switched to yoga from calisthenics after experimenting with a beginner's yoga class. You will find that the more you exercise, the

> # The more you exercise, the better you get to know your body, and this will help you to think of more variations to alleviate boredom.

better you will get to know your body, and this will help you think up more variations to alleviate boredom.

A New Type of Behavior

You are aiming for a type of behavior modification. You are trying gradually and slowly to mold yourself from a totally sedentary individual into a person who easily and readily takes part in a balanced exercise program consisting of aerobic, stretching, and strength-building routines.

This is by no means an easy task. During the first 6 to 8 weeks especially, you might hear a persistent internal voice urging you to give up. It's easy to listen to that voice. You will think of a million rationalizations for quitting. We suggest that when that voice whispers the reasons why you should quit, you should respond with the reasons to keep going and try to remember that the first 6 to 8 weeks are by far the hardest.

Things will get a lot easier as your cardiovascular system increases in capacity, your muscles get stronger, and your body becomes more flexible. You may even experience "runner's high," a feeling of euphoria that some runners claim they get after running for long periods of time. Or you may never experience any type of euphoria. But we can promise that you will feel stronger and more confident while you are exercising and between sessions. If you follow the guidelines in this book, you will feel mental and physical benefits that should give you all the incentive you need to continue your exercises.

Consider the words of David A. Field, who began exercising regularly when he was 45 years old in 1963. By 1981, after averaging about 950 miles a year, running an average of 268

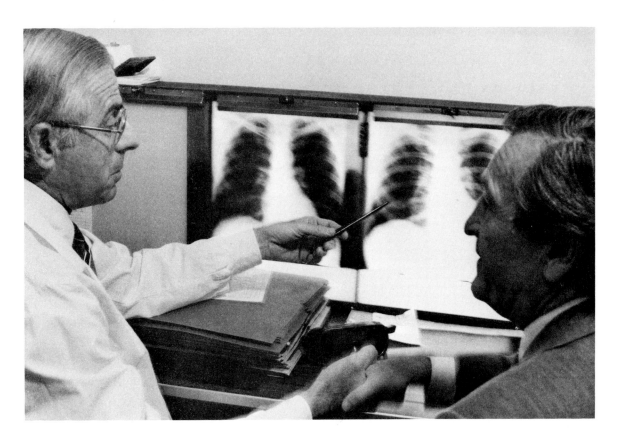

days a year, Field discovered that he had made considerable improvements in his physical conditioning. Nevertheless, what mattered most to him, he wrote, was the following: "As long as the daily workout remains fun I will continue. . . . My workouts helped me to be very aware of the beauty around me: the warm weather that follows a winter that has remained too long, a crisp fall that follows a sweltering summer. All have made daily exercise well worth my time."[6]

Perhaps the final words belong to Dr. Cooper, writing about the difficulties and rewards of getting through the first 6 to 8 weeks: "Once you're past that period, I can promise that you'll begin to enjoy your workout. After eight to ten weeks, you sense the change. You'll find yourself looking forward to your exercise, longing for it as an accustomed pleasure."

[6] David A. Field, *The Physician and Sportsmedicine*, April 1981, p. 143.

ACKNOWLEDGMENTS

Page 2, "The Fitness Mania," *U.S. News & World Report*, February 27, 1978. Reprinted by permission of *U.S. News & World Report*.

Pages 3, 27–28, from *The Whole Heart Book* by James J. Nora, M.D., M.P.H. Copyright © 1980 by James Jackson Nora. Reprinted by permission of Holt, Rinehart and Winston, Publishers.

Page 4, "A Very Simple Guide to Help You Feel Better," 1980. Reprinted by permission of Blue Cross/Blue Shield Associations.

Page 6, Ralph S. Paffenbarger, Jr. et al., "Current Exercise and Heart Attack Risk," *Cardiac Rehabilitation*, Summer 1979. Reprinted by permission of *Cardiac Rehabilitation*, an affiliate of the American Heart Association.

Pages 6–7, Robert S. Eliot et al., "The Physician in the Work Setting," *The American Journal of Cardiology*, March 1981. Reprinted by permission of *The American Journal of Cardiology*.

Page 10, Joseph LaDou, *The Executive*, March 1979. Reprinted by permission of *The Executive*, Cornell University Graduate School of Business and Public Administration.

Pages 16, 31, 56–57, 158, James F. Fixx, *The Complete Book of Running*. Copyright © 1977 by Random House, Inc. Reprinted by permission of Random House, Inc.

Pages 16, 57, 58–60, *Guidelines for Successful Jogging*, published by the American Running and Fitness Association (formerly the National Jogging Association), Washington, D.C. Reprinted by permission of the American Running and Fitness Association.

Page 16, reprinted from the November 7, 1977 issue of *Business Week* by special permission, copyright © 1977 by McGraw-Hill, Inc., New York, N.Y. 10020. All rights reserved.

Page 17, Bernard L. Gladieux, Jr., *Running & Fitness* (formerly *The Jogger*), published by the American Running and Fitness Association (formerly the National Jogging Association), Washington, D.C. Reprinted by permission of the American Running and Fitness Association.

Pages 17, 27, 131, from *The Aerobics Way* by Kenneth H. Cooper, M.D., M.P.H. Copyright © 1977 by Kenneth H. Cooper. Reprinted by permission of the publisher, M. Evans and Company, Inc., 216 East 49 St., New York, N.Y. 10017.

Page 21, "Before You Begin an Exercise Program," adapted from American College of Sports Medicine, *Guidelines for Graded Exercise Testing and Exercise Prescription*, 2d ed., Lea & Febiger, Philadelphia, 1980. By permission of Lea & Febiger.

Pages 34, 45, 152, from *Aerobics* by Kenneth H. Cooper, M.D., M.P.H. Copyright © 1968 by Kenneth H. Cooper and Kevin Brown. Reprinted by permission of the publisher, M. Evans and Company, Inc., 216 East 49 St., New York, N.Y. 10017.

Pages 44, 68, 152, Lenore R. Zohman, M.D., Albert A. Kattus, M.D., and Donald G. Softness, *The Cardiologists' Guide to Fitness and Health through Exercise*. Copyright © 1979 by Lenore R. Zohman, M.D., Albert A. Kattus, M.D., and Donald G. Softness. Reprinted by permission of Simon & Schuster, a division of Gulf & Western Corporation.

Page 46, Rudolph H. Dressendorfer, "Endurance Training of Recreationally Active Men," reprinted from *The Physician and Sportsmedicine*, November 1978, a McGraw-Hill publication.

Pages 51–54, Charles T. Kuntzleman, *The Complete Book of Walking*, 1979. Reprinted by permission of Publications International Ltd.

Page 52, Yehuda Shoenfeld, M.D., et al., "Walking: A Method for Rapid Improvement of Physical Fitness," *Journal of the American Medical Association*, May 23, 1980. Copyright © 1980, American Medical Association. Reprinted by permission of the American Medical Association.

Pages 63–64, J. Thomas Bohlmann, "Injuries in Competitive Cycling," reprinted from *The Physician and Sportsmedicine*, May 1981, a McGraw-Hill publication.

Page 66, Eugene A. Sloan, *The Complete Book of Bicycling*. Copyright © 1970 by Eugene A. Sloan. Reprinted by permission of Simon & Schuster, a division of Gulf & Western Corporation.

Page 71, Bud Getchell, Ph.D., and Pat Clearly, M.A., "The Caloric Costs of Rope Skipping and Running," reprinted from *The Physician and Sportsmedicine*, February 1980, a McGraw-Hill publication.

Page 133, by permission of Richard O. Keelor.

Page 134, Jack Martin, "The New Business Boom—Employee Fitness," *Nation's Business*, February 1978. Reprinted by permission of *Nation's Business*.

Pages 137, 138–139, Dennis Colacino, Roy Larsen, Keith Fogle, and Curtis S. Wilbur, reprinted from *The Physician and Sportsmedicine*, May 1980, a McGraw-Hill publication.

Page 137, Malcolm Forbes, *Newsweek*, May 23, 1977, p. 79. Reprinted by permission of *Newsweek*.

Pages 139–140, article by Bob Glover reprinted with permission from *Running & Fitness*, official publication of the American Running and Fitness Association, Washington, D.C. Copyright © 1981 by the American Running and Fitness Association. All rights reserved.

Pages 149–150, George A. Bray, M.D., quoted in Jane Brody, *The New York Times*, February 24, 1981. Copyright © 1981 by The New York Times Company. Reprinted by permission.

Pages 154–155, Dr. Jean Mayer, *Project Health: Gift of Energy*. Reprinted by permission of G.D. Searle & Company.

Page 156, Theodore Van Itallie, M.D., quoted in R. Lewin, "Overblown Reports Distort Obesity Risks," *Science*, Vol. 211, January 16, 1981. Copyright © 1981 by the American Association for the Advancement of Science. Reprinted by permission.

Pages 159–160, Joseph J. Morella and Richard J. Turchetti, *Nutrition and the Athlete*, 1976. Reprinted by permission of Mason-Charter.

Page 170, Margaret Dunkle, "What Constitutes Equality for Women in Sports," September 1975. Reprinted by permission of the Project on the Status and Education of Women.

Page 171, Letha Yurko Hunter, "The Female Athlete," *Medical Times*, June 1981. Reprinted by permission of *Medical Times*.

Page 172, by permission of Dorothy Harris.

Pages 172–173, Joan Gillette, quoted in *The Washington Post*, June 27, 1976. Reprinted by permission of The Associated Press.

Page 173, 174, Mona Shangold, M.D., *Running & Fitness* (formerly *The Jogger*), November-December 1980, published by the American Running and Fitness Association (formerly the National Jogging Association), Washington, D.C. Reprinted by permision of the American Running and Fitness Association.

Page 176, John P. O'Shea and Julie Wegner, "Power Weight Training and the Female Athlete," reprinted from *The Physician and Sportsmedicine*, June 1981, a McGraw-Hill publication.

Page 176, Ruth Weeks, M.D., quoted in *Working Woman*, January 1980. Reprinted by permission of *Working Woman*.

Page 177, Dr. Suzanne Hayes and Dr. Manning Feinleib, *American Journal of Public Health*, Vol. 70, No. 2, February 1980. Reprinted by permission of Dr. Suzanne Hayes, Dr. Manning Feinleib, and the American Public Health Association.

Page 177, Stanford University study reprinted from *The Washington Post*, January 8, 1981. Reprinted by permission of United Press International.

Page 177, Irvin H. Gracer quoted in Jane Adams, *Woman on Top*, Hawthorn Books, N.Y. Copyright © 1979 by E.P. Dutton, Inc. Reprinted by permission of E.P. Dutton, Inc.

Page 184, Robert Kerlan, M.D., quoted in Sally Ogle Davis, "The Battle of Wounded Knees," *The New York Times Magazine*, December 7, 1980. Copyright © 1980 by The New York Times Company. Reprinted by permission.

Page 185, Philip A. Witman et al., "Common Problems Seen in a Metropolitan Sports Clinic," reprinted from *The Physician and Sportsmedicine*, March 1981, a McGraw-Hill publication.

Pages 190, 191, Robert C. Cantu, *Toward Fitness*, Human Sciences Press, 1980. Reprinted by permission of Human Sciences Press.

Page 192, Erika S. Sivarajan et al., *The New England Journal of Medicine*, Vol. 305, No. 1, pp. 357–362. Reprinted by permission of *The New England Journal of Medicine*.

Pages 192–193, Thomas M. Flood, "Ten Steps To a Successful Exercise Program," *Medical Times*, May 1980. Reprinted by permission of *Medical Times*.

Page 194, Alan R. Morton et al., reprinted from *The Physician and Sportsmedicine*, March 1981, a McGraw-Hill publication.

Page 194, Dr. Richard E. Winter, "Low Back Pain: Its Control & Prevention," *Over 40*, November 1978. Reprinted by permission of Dr. Richard E. Winter.

Page 198, David A. Field, reprinted from *The Physician and Sportsmedicine*, April 1981, a McGraw-Hill publication.

Page 198, from *The New Aerobics* by Kenneth H. Cooper, M.D., M.P.H. Copyright © 1970 by Kenneth H. Cooper. Reprinted by permission of the publisher, M. Evans and Company, Inc., 216 East 49 St., New York, N.Y. 10017.

INDEX

Heart (*Cont.*):
    oxygen supply to, 33–34
        (*See also* Aerobics)
    (*See also* Pulse taking; Target zone)
Heart attacks, 5–6, 8
    ameliorating risk factors for, 9–13
    economic costs of, 134
    employee fitness program in prevention of, 133
    exercise following, 51, 189–192
    obesity and, 156
    sedentary lifestyle and, 1, 2
Heartbeat (*see* Pulse taking; Target zone)
Heel injuries, 51, 185
Helmets for bicycling, 182
High-risk intervention program of Pepsico, 137
Hip problems, walking with, 51
Hormones, role of, in muscle development, 170, 175
Hot showers after exercising, 127, 131
Hunter, Letha Yurko, 171
Hypertension, 190, 195
    as controllable risk factor, 9, 10
    effects of weight loss on, 166
    sedentary lifestyle and, 4
    strength-building exercises contraindicated with, 75
    walking with, 52

Ice skating, 39
Ideal weight, 157
Indoor cycling, 24, 40–42, 61, 62, 65
    alleviating boredom of, 41–42, 196
    footwear for, 181
Industrial society, reduced physical exertion in, 1–3, 5
Information sources:
    on employee fitness programs, 136, 146
    on walking, 53
Injuries, 75, 179–187
    arthritis and joint, 193
    incurred with strength-building exercises, 75
    most common, 184, 185
    overstraining and permanent, 50
    postpartum, 173
    prevention of, 183–187
        (*See also* Clothing; Footwear)
    due to tight muscles, 94
        (*See also* Yoga exercises)
    (*See also specific types of injuries*)
Intensity of exercise, 23, 26
International Journal of Obesity (magazine), 149
Isometrics, 19, 25, 75–83
    abdominal, 81
    for arm muscles, 80
    for buttocks, 82, 140

Isometrics (*Cont.*):
    cardiovascular disease and, 76
    for chest muscles, 81
    for leg muscles, 65, 83
    for neck muscles, 78
    right time for, 30, 31
    for thighs and lower back, 82
    upper-body, 79
    at work, 140
    (*See also* Calisthenics; Strength-building exercises; Weight lifting)
Isotonics, 19, 25
    during aerobics cooling-down period, 83, 84, 91, 92
    for leg muscles, 65
    (*See also* Calisthenics; Strength-building exercises; Weight lifting)

James Richardson & Sons fitness program, 136
Jogger's kidney (athletic pseudonephritis), 186
Jogging, 15, 24, 54–61
    basis for selecting, 38, 39
    beginner's program for, 57–61
    calories used per mile of, 55
    clothing for, 181–182
    effects of, on cardiovascular system, 45
    in employee fitness programs, 135
    right time for, 29, 31
    running vs., 16–17
        (*See also* Running)
    shoes for, 180–181
    warming-up and cooling-down periods with, 60, 126–128
    weight loss with, 159–161
Johns Manville fitness program, 136
Johnson&Johnson fitness program, 133
Joint injuries, 193
    (*See also injuries to specific joints*)
Jumping (*see* Rope skipping)
Jumping jacks, 39–41, 83

Katz, Jane, 70
Kavanaugh, Terence, 190–191
Keelor, Richard O., 3, 133
Kerlan, Robert, 184
Kimberly-Clark fitness program, 133, 135, 136
Knee injuries, 51, 62, 179, 184, 185
Knee lifts at work, 144
Kuntzleman, Charles T., 51, 53, 54

LaDou, Joseph, 10
Larsen, Roy, 138

Running (*Cont.*):
   swimming compared with, 67
   walking combined with, 55–56, 58–60
   walking compared with, 51
   warming-up and cooling-down periods with, 60, 126–128
   weight loss with, 159–160
Running Times (magazine), 180
Ryan, Alan J., 17

Salt intake, need to reduce, 5, 158
Salute to the sun, exercise, 95, 102–108, 130
Saunas:
   in employee fitness program, 135
   following exercise, 127, 131
Scaff, Jack, 191
Scarsdale diet, 149
Seat adjustment on bicycles, 63–64
Sedentary lifestyle, 3–6, 34
   and cardiac rehabilitation, 190
   as controllable risk factor, 9, 10
   degenerative effects of, 3, 4
   exercise as antidote to, 4–6
      (*See also* Exercise regimen; *specific types of exercise*)
Sex as uncontrollable risk factor, 9, 10
Sexual activity, effects of exercise on, 13
Shangold, Mona, 170, 173, 174
Share-cost employee fitness programs, 147
Shin splints, 51, 185
Shoes (*see* Footwear)
Shorter, Frank, 16, 37
Shoulder injuries, 184
Shoulder stands, exercise, 111–112
Showers, hot, following exercise, 127, 131
Sickness (*see* Disease and disability)
Side stretches, 128
Situps, 85, 93, 128, 131
   effects of, on abdominal muscles, 8, 19, 88
   frequency, duration, and intensity of, 25
   injuries incurred with, 75
Skating, 24, 39
Skiing, cross-country, 24, 38, 39, 43
Skipping (*see* Rope skipping)
Sloan, Eugene A., 66
Smith, Darwin E., 135
Smoking (*see* Cigarette smoking)
Sneakers (*see* Footwear)
Soccer, 39
Spinal twist, exercise, 122–124
Sports medicine, growth of, 183
Squash, 38, 39
   drawbacks of, 41, 43
   in employee fitness programs, 135, 136

Squash (*Cont.*):
   tennis compared with, 44
Stair climbing, 8, 30
   by cardiac patients, 191
   at work, 145–146
Standing leg stretches, 126–127
Steam room, using, following exercise, 127, 131
Stillman water diet, 149
Stomach muscles (*see* Abdominal muscles)
Strength, building reserve, with exercise, 11–13
Strength-building exercises, 18–19, 25, 197
   aerobics and: combined, 74, 92
      difference between, 74–75
   bicycling complemented with, 73
   clothing for, 183
   in cooling-down period, 126
   duration of, 26
   golf and, 43, 44
   injuries incurred with, 179, 185
   need for regular, 195
   (*See also* Calisthenics; Isometrics; Isotonics)
Stress and anxiety, 7, 13, 195
   coping with, 5, 12
   experienced by women executives, 176–177
   running or jogging to reduce, 55
      (*See also* Jogging; Running)
   and strength-building exercises, 74
      (*See also* Strength-building exercises)
   stress management programs in employee fitness programs, 135
   stretching exercises for, 94
      (*See also* Stretching exercises)
   walking for, 54, 57
      (*See also* Walking)
Stress leg fractures, 185
Stress test, 19–24, 26
   in employee fitness programs, 136, 137
   for rope skipping, 71
   for running or jogging, 55
Stretching exercises, 18, 24, 44, 49, 73, 93, 197
   for Achilles tendon and calf muscles, 127
   in automobiles, 30–31
   duration of, 26
   footwear for, 181
   injuries incurred with, 179
   for lower-back pain, 18, 194
   need for regular, 195
   purpose of, 94
      (*See also* Flexibility)
   swimming preceded by, 68
   warming up with, 49, 126
   at work, 143
   (*See also* Yoga exercises)